THE MRCS EXAMINATION:
MCQs AND EMQs

The MRCS Examination:
MCQs and EMQs

PAUL CHATRATH
MA (Cantab) MBBS (London) MRCS (Eng)
Addenbrooke's Hospital, Cambridge

OMAR RAHIM
BSc (Hons) MBBS (London) MRCS (Eng)
The Royal London Hospital, London

**Blackwell
Science**

© 1999 by Blackwell Science Ltd
Editorial Offices:
Osney Mead, Oxford OX2 0EL
25 John Street, London
WC1N 2BL
23 Ainslie Place, Edinburgh
EH3 6AJ
350 Main Street, Malden
MA 02148-5018, USA
54 University Street, Carlton
Victoria 3053, Australia
10, rue Casimir Delavigne
75006 Paris, France

Other Editorial Offices:
Blackwell Wissenschafts-Verlag GmbH
Kurfürstendamm 57
10707 Berlin, Germany

Blackwell Science KK
MG Kodenmacho Building
7–10 Kodenmacho Nihombashi
Chuo-ku, Tokyo 104, Japan

First Published 1999

Transferred to digital print 2005

Set by Bookcraft Ltd, Stroud
Printed and bound in Great Britain by
Marston Book Services Limited, Oxford

DISTRIBUTORS

Marston Book Services Ltd
PO Box 269
Abingdon, Oxon OX14 4YN
(*Orders*: Tel: 01235 465500
Fax: 01235 465555)

USA
Blackwell Science, Inc.
Commerce Place
350 Main Street
Malden, MA 02148-5018
(*Orders*: Tel: 800 759 6102
781 388 8250
Fax: 781 388 8255)

Canada
Login Brothers Book Company
324 Saulteaux Crescent
Winnipeg, Manitoba R3J 3T2
(*Orders*: Tel: 204 837 2987)

Australia
Blackwell Science Pty Ltd
54 University Street
Carlton, Victoria 3053
(*Orders*: Tel: 3 9347 0300
Fax: 3 9347 5001)

A catalogue record for this title is
available from the British Library

ISBN 0-632-05402-6

Library of Congress Cataloging-in-Publication
Data

Chatrath, Paul.
The MRCS examination: MCQs and EMQs/
Paul Chatrath & Omar Rahim.
p.   cm.
ISBN 0-632-05402-6
1. Surgery Examinations, questions, etc.
I. Rahim, Omar. II. Title.
RD37.2.C47 1999
617'.0076—dc21
DNLM/DLC
for Library of Congress   99-35373
CIP

For further information on
Blackwell Science, visit our website:
www.blackwell-science.com

Contents

Preface

This book is intended primarily for use by those studying for the written papers of the MRCS/AFRCS examinations. The authors have recently obtained their Membership of The Royal College of Surgeons and have first hand experience of the style of questions used and the standard required. The book contains 250 multiple choice questions and 30 extended matching questions which have been chosen to reflect the balance between basic science topics and clinical subjects which appears in the exam. Extensive explanations are also included. The format of the book closely mirrors that of the distance learning course provided by The Royal College of Surgeons of England. The book will also be of use to medical students studying for Finals as an additional source of surgical questions.

Structure of the
MRCS Written Papers

There are two written papers, one covering the **Core** modules and one the **Systems** modules. Each paper lasts 2 hours and contains approximately 45 multiple choice questions (MCQs) and 20 to 30 extended matching questions (EMQs). In the written papers for the MRCS (Eng) there is no negative marking. This means that it is good technique to answer all the questions even if you are not sure you are right. In 1998 the AFRCS examination used negative marking.

MCQs

Each question has a common stem and on average 5 statements, although the exact number of statements may vary for each question. The answer to each statement may be either true or false. A mark is awarded for a correct answer to the statement, whether it is true or false.

EMQs

Each question begins with a list of possible options, and is followed by several case histories or statements which must be matched with the correct option from the list. There may be more than one option from the list which apply to the given statement but the answer is the one which *best* applies. A mark is given for each correct answer.

How to use this book

This book is divided into **Core** and **Systems** sections, each of which contains five separate modules. Each module is composed of 25 multiple choice questions and 3 extended matching questions, which are followed by extensive explanations.

The questions in each section are based on material which appears in the corresponding module of the distance learning course run by The Royal College of Surgeons of England. This makes it easy for students to test themselves on each module in turn as they work through or revise the course. However the book is also well suited to being used in its own right at the end of a period of revision, such as in the weeks before the exam itself.

Section 1
Core Modules

1: Perioperative Management 1

1 In general anaesthesia:
A Ketamine should be avoided in the haemodynamically shocked patient
B Hyperkalaemia is a recognized side effect of suxamethonium
C Etomidate is less depressant on the myocardium than other general anaesthetic agents
D Sellick's manoeuvre should be avoided in pregnant women
E Thiopentone is the drug of choice in day-case anaesthesia

2 Local anaesthetics:
A The maximum adult dose of lignocaine with adrenaline is 300 mg
B Bupivacaine has a faster onset and longer duration of action than lignocaine
C Bupivacaine is the drug of choice for a Bier's block
D The occurrence of a vasovagal attack is an indication of toxicity
E The higher the pKa of an agent, the faster its onset of action

3 Preoperatively, an ECG should be requested in:
A All patients over the age of 50
B Diabetics
C Patients undergoing carpal tunnel decompression
D Patients on digoxin therapy
E Afro-Caribbeans

4 Appropriate investigations for a 62-year-old Indian man undergoing transhiatal oesophago-gastrectomy include:
A HIV test
B Exercise ECG test
C Chest X-ray
D Spirometry
E Sickle-cell screen

5 Ultrasound is the investigation of choice in:
A Cystic breast masses
B Right upper quadrant abdominal pain
C Intra-abdominal bleeding
D Breast screening of patients aged 50–64
E Bone metastases

6 Pulse oximetry:
A Measures the adequacy of tissue oxygen delivery
B Is affected by ambient light
C Has lower values in the presence of carboxyhaemoglobinaemia
D Has higher values in the presence of nail varnish
E Is inaccurate below values of 85%

7 Regarding surgery in diabetics:
A There is an increased incidence of postoperative wound dehiscence
B Insulin sliding scales are routinely continued into the intraoperative period
C There is an increased incidence of myocardial infarction perioperatively
D A BM Stix should be done every hour during the first postoperative day
E Patients are best treated by day-case surgery when appropriate

8 Patients with chronic obstructive airways disease:

A Should not undergo elective surgery during the summer months

B Typically receive perioperative prophylactic antibiotics

C Must never receive more than 21% oxygen

D Nonsteroidal anti-inflammatory drugs are the postoperative analgesics of first choice

E Who stop smoking the day before surgery have a reduced operative mortality

9 A patient with a haemoglobin of 11 g/L:

A Preoperatively should receive a blood transfusion

B Has a markedly reduced tissue oxygenation

C Has an increased risk of perioperative myocardial infarction

D Postoperatively should receive an immediate blood transfusion if short of breath

E Is at greater risk in the presence of co-existing ischaemic heart disease

10 The following may be of value in patients with ischaemic heart disease:

A A thallium scan

B Spirometry

C A chest X-ray

D Ensuring sufficient hypervolaemia intraoperatively

E Stopping smoking 12 hours preoperatively

11 Regarding elderly patients undergoing major surgery:

A Low molecular weight heparin is the preferred agent for thromboembolic prophylaxis

B There is a lower incidence of deep venous thrombosis when above knee rather than below knee compression stockings are used

C Deep venous thromboses are treated with unfractionated heparin only

D Fluid depletion increases the risk of deep venous thrombosis

E The period of postoperative bed rest is commonly prolonged when receiving heparin

12 Obese patients:

A Tend to present earlier with appendicitis than in non-obese individuals

B Are more likely to develop incisional hernias

C Have an increased risk of wound dehiscence

D Have a higher rate of infection with *Staphylococcus aureus*

E Should not undergo laparoscopic surgery

13 In patients with jaundice:

A Of hepatocellular aetiology, an abnormal prothrombin time should respond to intramuscular vitamin K

B Mannitol is used if the urine output is low

C Excess unconjugated bilirubin is usually associated with dark urine

D ERCP is the investigation of choice in the presence of painful jaundice

E The INR is commonly decreased

14 The following relate to HIV positive and AIDS patients:

A Needlestick injuries with a solid needle are associated with a higher risk of transmission of the HIV virus than with a hollow needle

B Elective hernia repair is classified as a clean operation

C Prophylactic use of AZT is mandatory

D Anorectal surgery is contraindicated in AIDS patients

E Mycobacterial infection or lymphoma complicated by a perforated intra-abdominal viscus is a strong indication for laparotomy

15 Causes of immunosuppression include:

A Severe jaundice

B Hypergammaglobulinaemia

C Myelofibrosis

D Blood transfusion

E Hypoxia

16 **The following are associated with an increased risk of deep venous thrombosis:**
A Smoking
B Thrombocytopaenia
C Buerger's disease
D Cardiac failure
E Intraoperative head up table tilt

17 **The following appear blue on a Gram stain:**
A Bacillus
B Diphtheroids
C *Proteus*
D *Yersinia enterocolitica*
E *Neisseria meningitidis*

18 **Sequelae of streptococcal infections include:**
A Rheumatic fever
B Glomerulonephritis
C Meningitis
D Liver abscess
E Erysipelas

19 **Diathermy:**
A Of the bipolar type requires the use of a patient electrode
B Has a current of 400 Hz
C The patient electrode should be greater than 70 cm^2
D Accidental burns are characteristically partial thickness
E Of the monopolar type is generally safer than bipolar

20 **Methods of sterilization of theatre instruments and equipment include:**
A Ethylene oxide
B 2% glutaraldehyde
C Laminar air flow
D Chlorhexidine
E Steam and/or pressure

21 *Escherichia coli:*
A Is Gram negative and non-motile
B Is a commensal of the alimentary tract
C May cause wound infection
D May cause meningitis
E Commonly causes postoperative pneumonia in smokers

22 **The following methods reduce postoperative wound infection:**
A Laminar air flow
B The use of a face mask by the surgeon
C Theatre clothing
D A plastic adhesive drape over the operation site
E Blood transfusion

23 **Hepatitis B:**
A Is an RNA virus
B Has an incubation period of 4 to 6 weeks
C Antibodies to C-antigen are indicative of carrier status
D Is less infectious than HIV
E Is transmitted by the faeco-oral route

24 **The following suture materials are absorbable:**
A Polydioxanone
B Polyglactin
C Dexon
D Prolene
E Nylon

25 **Spinal anaesthesia:**
A Is contraindicated in patients with multiple sclerosis
B Has a slower onset of action than epidural anaesthesia
C Hypotension is less common than with epidural anaesthesia
D Produces a light motor block
E Is rarely associated with a dural tap

EXTENDED MATCHING QUESTIONS

Topic: Drug interactions

A Glyceryl trinitrate
B Thyroxine
C Cisplatin
D Captopril
E Micronor
F Atenolol
G Frusemide
H Heparin
I Prednisolone

For each side effect, select the most likely causative drug from the list of options above. Each option may be used once, more than once or not at all.

1 Marrow suppression
2 Adrenal suppression
3 Hyperkalaemia
4 Ototoxicity

Topic: Infections

A *Staphylococcus aureus*
B *Candida albicans*
C *Yersinia*
D *Klebsiella*
E *Pseudomonas aeruginosa*
F *Clostridium perfringens*
G *Brucella melitensis*

For each clinical diagnosis, select the most likely causative organism from the list of options above. Each option may be used once, more than once or not at all.

1 Oesophagitis
2 Appendicitis
3 Urinary tract infection
4 Burn complicated by infection
5 Bronchiectasis

Topic: Antibiotics

A Benzylpenicillin
B Chloramphenicol
C Cefuroxime
D Metronidazole
E Tetracycline
F Clindamycin

For each clinical situation, select the most appropriate antibiotic from the list of options above. Each option may be used once, more than once or not at all.

1 Appendicitis
2 Otitis media
3 *Clostridium perfringens* infection
4 Prophylaxis for a total hip replacement

ANSWERS TO MULTIPLE CHOICE QUESTIONS

1 In general anaesthesia:
A False
B True
C True
D False
E False

Ketamine is often used in patients who are hypovolaemic although its side effects include hallucinations and mental problems. **Etomidate** is used for induction of anaesthesia and has the advantage of maintaining cardiac output. **Suxamethonium** is a depolarising muscle relaxant, and its side effects include histamine release, bradycardia, hyperkalaemia, persistent blockade and malignant hyperthermia. **Sellick's manoeuvre** is the application of cricoid pressure resulting in occlusion of the oesophagus against the fixed vertebral column posteriorly. It is advised in pregnant women in order to protect against aspiration. **Thiopentone** has been replaced by propofol which has a very short half-life, and which is the preferred agent for day-case surgery.

2 Local anaesthetics:
A False
B False
C False
D False
E False

A total dose of 300 mg of lignocaine may be safely used in an adult, but this may be increased to 500 mg when combined with adrenaline. Bupivacaine has a higher pKa than lignocaine and therefore a slower onset of action. It also has a longer duration of action and is often combined with lignocaine to produce local anaesthesia which is both fast acting and long lasting. Prilocaine is the drug of first choice for use in a Bier's block owing to its high therapeutic index. This means that toxicity is rarely a problem even if drug escape into the general circulation occurs. However, bupivacaine is associated with a significant risk of ventricular arrhythmias which precludes its safe use in Bier's block. Features of toxicity include perioral tingling, dizziness with slurred speech, and ultimately convulsions and coma.

3 Preoperatively, an ECG should be requested in:
A False
B True
C False
D True
E False

Current guidelines for requesting a preoperative ECG include patients over the age of 60 (although the precise age cut-off may vary from hospital to hospital), those with known cardiac disease or conditions with cardiac complications such as diabetes mellitus or hypertension, operations which have cardiac implications such as an Ivor Lewis repair, arrhythmogenic drugs such as digoxin, and if cardiac disease is suspected following clinical examination such as the finding of an irregular pulse. Carpal tunnel decompression by itself does not warrant an ECG, and Afro-Caribbean patients should be investigated for sickle-cell disease but do not have any increased risk of cardiac disease.

4 Appropriate investigations for a 62-year-old Indian man undergoing transhiatal oesophago-gastrectomy include:
A False
B False
C True
D True
E True

A 62-year-old Indian man undergoing transhiatal oesophago-gastrectomy should have a chest radiograph and spirometry in view of the nature of the surgery and potential thoracic complications. Asian patients have an increased risk of sickle-cell disease. An exercise ECG test is not indicated on the basis of the information given so far. The history should however be directed towards elucidating the risk factors for cardiac disease which has a higher incidence in Indian men at this age in the UK. Unless there is a definite suspicion of risk, routine testing of HIV is not required. If an HIV test is recommended, the patient should be encouraged to seek advice from a trained counsellor due to the implications of being tested, whether positive or negative.

5 Ultrasound is the investigation of choice in:
A True
B True
C False
D False
E False

Ultrasound is widely used in the investigation of biliary and urogenital disease as it takes advantage of the differences in echogenicity between neighbouring structures. This makes it useful in discriminating between solid and cystic masses, which is also of benefit in the investigation of breast disease. A discrete cystic breast mass is however probably best investigated with fine needle aspiration cytology. Mammography or plain radiography of the breast using high resolution films and X-rays are carried out as part of the breast screening programme in women between 50 and 64 years of age. Bone metastases may show up on plain radiography but an isotope bone scan may be required to detect smaller lesions. Following attention to resuscitation, intractable intra-abdominal bleeding should be investigated and treated by laparotomy although selective angiography may be indicated in specific situations.

6 Pulse oximetry:
A False
B True
C False
D False
E False

Pulse oximetry measures the arterial oxygen saturation of haemoglobin and *not* the adequacy of tissue oxygen delivery. The latter depends upon a number of other factors including cardiac output and the metabolic demands of the tissues. Ambient light and shivering may affect the readings obtained. Carboxyhaemoglobinaemia may arise secondary to carbon monoxide poisoning which can cause readings to tend artificially towards 100%. Nail varnish may result in misleadingly low values. Readings may be difficult to ascertain when patients are cold or peripherally vasoconstricted. A saturation of 70% is generally taken as the level below which readings are inaccurate.

7 Regarding surgery in diabetics:
A True
B False
C False
D False
E False

Caution must always be exercised with diabetic patients undergoing operations, and day-case surgery is best avoided owing to the potential for the development of specific diabetes-related complications. Non-insulin dependent diabetic patients usually omit their normal oral hypoglycaemic dose on the day of surgery, or earlier, depending on the duration of action of the agent which they take. Occasionally an insulin sliding scale regime may be required particularly for major surgery or poorly controlled blood sugar levels. The biggest danger to the anaesthetist and therefore to the patient is hypoglycaemia, especially that occurring intraoperatively, and so insulin tends not to be given during the operation. A BM Stix should be done every 4 hours after the operation, and in general the sooner patients are returned to their normal medication and diabetic control, the better. This will be related to the timing of commencement of oral feeding after the operation, which when back to normal will allow the restarting of the original thera-peutic regime. Patients with diabetes have an increased risk of sepsis, renal abnormalities and impaired wound healing.

8 **Patients with chronic obstructive airways disease:**
A False
B False
C False
D False
E True

Wherever possible elective surgery should take place during the months in which symptoms are least prominent, which for the majority of patients usually falls in the summer. Appropriate antibiotics should be prescribed for confirmed chest infections but are not given routinely for perioperative prophylaxis. The amount of oxygen that may be given to a patient with COAD causes concern to most medical staff. Such patients may rely on a hypoxic drive to breathing and if given too high a concentration of oxygen may develop respiratory failure. In general, all patients may be safely given O_2 in concentrations of 24–28% and if needed may be given a closely monitored trial with a higher oxygen concentration, using observations and arterial blood gas readings as a measure of response. Patients who are sensitive to aspirin should not be given non-steroidal anti-inflammatory analgesics as their pain can be adequately managed by the combined use of other simple analgesics, patient controlled devices (PCA), epidural, local and regional blocks. The effects of smoking on the cardiovascular system are mediated by carbon monoxide and nicotine. *Carbon monoxide* has a negative inotropic effect, and forms carboxyhaemoglobin which results in a marked left shift of the oxygen dissociation curve. *Nicotine* increases the heart rate and blood pressure. Both substances have half-lives of only a few hours; thus patients who stop smoking for at least 12 to 24 hours before surgery reduce the potential for cardiovascular complications. The

respiratory effects of smoking are increased mucus secretion, bronchoconstriction and worsening of ciliary clearance, although these effects take up to 6 weeks to improve after stopping smoking. Smokers are 6 times more likely to result in postoperative respiratory problems.

9 **A patient with a haemoglobin of 11 g/L:**
A False
B False
C False
D False
E True

Tissue oxygenation depends upon the cardiac output, blood viscosity, peripheral vascular resistance and oxygen carrying capacity of the blood. Maximal tissue oxygenation is achieved at a haemoglobin concentration of 11 g/L. In general, preoperative blood transfusion is not recommended but may be considered when the haemoglobin concentration falls below 10 g/L. Transfusion increases the patient's haematocrit and therefore blood viscosity, increases the circulating fluid volume, and delivers to the patient stored erythrocytes with a reduced oxygen carrying capacity. These problems may take several days to be overcome, thus any transfusion should ideally take place at least 48 hours before the operation. Other adverse effects include an increased risk of post-transfusion infection, and of deep vein thrombosis due to increased blood viscosity. Despite these concerns, a low haemoglobin may warrant transfusion in specific circumstances where an increase in oxygen delivery to the tissues is deemed essential. A good example is a patient with ischaemic heart disease with anaemia in whom an increase in cardiac work to meet the demands of the tissues may precipitate an acute coronary event. A postoperative haemoglobin of 11 g/L by itself is not usually an indication for transfusion, and shortness of breath in this context should be assessed and investigated thoroughly before being assumed to be secondary to anaemia.

10 The following may be of value in patients with ischaemic heart disease:

A True
B False
C True
D False
E True

A patient with ischaemic heart disease will require appropriate preoperative assessment including the necessary investigations such as an ECG exercise test or a thallium scan where necessary. It is important to remember that between one-quarter to one-half of patients with proven ischaemic heart disease will have a normal resting ECG. Patients with poor left ventricular function will need to be managed carefully in the perioperative period, and hypotension, hypoxia and fluid overload will need to be anticipated and avoided. As mentioned above, cessation of smoking as little as 12 hours preoperatively will have beneficial effects on improving cardiovascular function.

11 Regarding elderly patients undergoing major surgery:

A True
B False
C False
D True
E False

Deep venous thromboses (DVT) occur in up to one-quarter of surgical patients and one-half of orthopaedic patients in the absence of prophylaxis. Pulmonary emboli occur in 1–2% of these patients. Unfractionated heparin may be used as prophylaxis and in the treatment of DVTs. However, low molecular weight heparin has been associated with less perioperative bleeding and is as effective in the prevention of DVT and pulmonary embolism. It can also be used for the treatment of DVTs, which avoids the need for monitoring the APTT. Fluid depletion increases viscosity and will therefore increase the risk of DVTs. Despite the use of heparin, earlier mobilization of patients is the key to reducing the incidence of these complications. Research into the difference between above knee compared with below knee stockings has not been conclusive. Despite the theoretical advantages of above knee compression stockings, their use has been complicated by problems with fitting, and the tendency of stockings to roll down the leg produces constrictions.

12 Obese patients:

A False
B True
C True
D True
E False

Obesity presents diagnostic difficulties to the surgeon, with delayed presentation of many conditions, including appendicitis and perforation, due to the masking of signs. Such patients are also more likely to have other co-existing medical problems and have an increased risk of postoperative complications including deep venous thrombosis, atelectasis, haematoma, infection, dehiscence and incisional hernia. Laparoscopic surgery is often technically easier than open surgery in obese patients, and results in a smaller incision in many operations.

13 In patients with jaundice:

A False
B True
C False
D False
E False

Jaundiced patients require particular attention to specific aspects of their management. This is because they are at an increased risk of hepatic impairment, impaired clotting, infection, renal failure and venous thrombosis. The following factors need to be considered:

• *Preoperatively*   Avoid morphine in the pre-medication, insert a urinary catheter,

mannitol 1 hour before surgery, renal dose dopamine if required.
• *Intraoperatively* Give 0.9% saline to match the urine output (measured hourly), mannitol if required.
• *Postoperatively* Continue fluid administration for maintenance and to replace losses, mannitol if the urine output falls, measure U&E's daily.

The prothrombin time may be increased in patients with obstructive jaundice due to deficiency of the production of the vitamin K dependent clotting factors. However, decreased prothrombin synthesis caused by hepatocellular disease does not respond to intramuscular vitamin K. It is the conjugated bilirubin in obstructive jaundice that results in dark urine. ERCP is indicated in patients with jaundice that have dilated intra- or extra-hepatic bile ducts, and not necessarily in all cases of painful jaundice.

14 The following relate to HIV positive and AIDS patients:

A False
B True
C False
D False
E False

Hollow needles carry a greater risk of HIV transmission than solid ones when involved in needlestick injuries. A hernia repair involves an incision through non-infected skin under controlled clean circumstances, and is therefore classified as a clean operation. It does however remind us that outcome after an operation is dependent on a number of factors including the condition of the patient and any immunocompromised state. Anorectal surgery is the commonest form of surgery undertaken in HIV positive patients. The prognosis in patients with mycobacterial infection or lymphoma is extremely poor and therefore surgery is not recommended although it may be carried out in the event of an acute abdomen.

15 Causes of immunosuppression include:

A True
B False
C True
D True
E True

Causes of **immunosuppression** are classified into those which are *congenital* such as hypogammaglobulinaemia, and those which are *acquired* including trauma, leukaemia, myelofibrosis, drug-induced aplastic anaemia, splenectomy, HIV, steroids and other immunosuppressants, medical disorders, malignancy, hypoxia and blood transfusion.

16 The following are associated with an increased risk of deep vein thrombosis:

A False
B False
C True
D True
E True

The surgeon must be aware of those patients who are at an increased risk of developing postoperative deep venous thromboses. **Virchow's triad** describes the properties of the vessel wall, blood flow and blood constituents as factors involved in the formation of a thrombosis. Common risk factors include a previous DVT, malignancy, immobility, oral contraceptive pill, obesity, cardiac failure, myocardial infarction, vasculitis, pregnancy and hyperviscosity states. Smokers paradoxically have a lower incidence of DVT. Intraoperative immobility of the patient together with venous pooling of blood especially in the head-up position has also been suggested as a causal factor.

17 The following appear blue on a Gram stain:

A True
B True
C False
D False
E False

The **Gram stain** aids in the identification of bacteria. A positive Gram reaction is staining to give a blue colour, whereas a negative Gram stain is pink. This occurs because of the differences in composition of the cell wall. Initially both types of bacteria absorb the crystal violet stain. Since Gram negative bacteria have a high lipid content of their cell walls, the decolouriser ethanol is able to dissolve this and release the crystal violet stain. In Gram positive organisms, the decolouriser is unable to act as a solvent thus the crystal violet stain remains.

18 Sequelae of streptococcal infections include:
A True
B True
C True
D True
E True

Group A **streptococci** are common pathogens and result in skin and wound infections such as erysipelas, impetigo, tonsillitis and septicaemia. Rheumatic fever and acute glomerulonephritis are late complications of infection. *S. pneumoniae* causes pneumonia, otitis media, meningitis and septicaemia. *S. viridans* is associated with endocarditis. Abscesses in the liver and elsewhere may be formed by *S. milleri*.

19 Diathermy:
A False
B False
C True
D False
E False

Surgical diathermy involves the passage of high frequency alternating current through body tissue. Intense local concentration of current results in the generation of heat of up to 1000 °C. The current frequencies used range from 400 kHz to 10 MHz, considerably higher than the relatively low frequencies found in mains electricity (50 Hz) and of the threshold required to produce neuromuscular stimulation. Diathermy may be monopolar or bipolar, the latter using considerably less power with no need for a plate electrode as current passes between the two limbs of the hand-held forceps. Thus it is inherently safer than the monopolar type although no cutting can be done. In monopolar diathermy, the plate needs to have a good contact of at least 70 cm^2 to ensure as low a current density as possible, otherwise heating at this site will occur resulting in burns which are usually full thickness in nature.

20 Methods of sterilization of theatre instruments and equipment include:
A True
B False
C False
D False
E True

Sterilization is strictly defined as the removal of *all* microorganisms including spores and viruses, but in practice is taken to mean reduction in contamination down to one in a million organisms. Sterilization may be by steam under pressure, hot air, ethylene oxide, low-temperature steam and formaldehyde and irradiation. Glutaraldehyde is widely used as a *disinfectant* in the decontamination of flexible endoscopes, being active in reducing the number of some viable organisms but unable to eliminate all viruses and spores.

21 *Escherichia coli*:
A False
B True
C False
D True
E False

Escherichia coli (*E. coli*) is a Gram negative motile organism which is a normal commensal of the gastrointestinal tract. It is a facultative anaerobe. It causes urinary tract infections, neonatal meningitis (especially during the first 2 months following ascending maternal infection *in utero* or during birth), and gastroenteritis. The latter is due to a variety of subtypes each of which has slightly different effects. *Enterotoxigenic E. coli (ETEC)* causes traveller's diarrhoea, *enteroinvasive E. coli (EIEC)* produces a shigella-like illness and *enterohaemorrhagic E. coli (EHEC)* produces a severe form of haemorrhagic colitis. Postoperative pulmonary aspiration may lead to pneumonia secondary to bowel organisms such as *E. coli*, although this is not known to occur with increased frequency in smokers.

22 The following methods reduce postoperative wound infection:
A True
B False
C False
D False
E False

Many of the methods used to control infection are theoretical; they may reduce the amount of bacteria in the wound but have not been shown to reduce the incidence of infection. There is little evidence to prove that infection is reduced by the use of face masks, theatre clothing or adhesive drapes. Laminar air flow has been shown to reduce infection, and is particularly employed in orthopaedic implant surgery. Blood transfusion has some immunosuppressive effects and may thereby increase infection.

23 Hepatitis B:
A False
B False
C False
D False
E False

Hepatitis B is a DNA virus which is spread by blood products, secretions, and sexual intercourse. The incubation period is 1 to 6 months, after which hepatitis B surface antigen (sAg) is detectable. In 5–10% of patients, this persists after 6 months resulting in the development of the carrier state. During the acute illness, IgM antibodies to hepatitis cAg are present in high titre and IgG antibodies in moderate titre. After the acute illness, persistent IgG antibodies to cAg imply previous infection. The presence of hepatitis B 'e' antigen (eAg) indicates high infectivity and is usually present for 1 to 3 months after the acute illness. The presence of antibodies to hepatitis B eAg indicates low infectivity.

24 The following suture materials are absorbable:
A True
B True
C True
D False
E False

PDS is polydioxanone and vicryl is polyglactin.

25 Spinal anaesthesia:
A True
B False
C False
D False
E False

Spinal anaesthesia provides effective and rapid blockade, but is more likely to result in hypotension and a more dense motor block than epidural anaesthesia. It is a one-off procedure compared with epidural anaesthesia in which a catheter may be left *in situ*. A much smaller dose of anaesthetic is used in spinal blocks, and consequently the duration of anaesthesia is in general shorter than with epidurals. The dura is routinely punctured when a spinal needle is inserted into the correct anatomical position, unlike with epidural insertion in which the catheter should lie in the extradural space. Consequently the incidence of post-dural headaches is higher following spinal than epidural anaesthesia. Contraindications to epidural and spinal blocks include bleeding disorders, sepsis and neurological disease.

ANSWERS TO EXTENDED MATCHING QUESTIONS

Topic: Drug interactions

1 C
2 I
3 D
4 C

Topic: Infections

1 B
2 C

3 D
4 A
5 E

Topic: Antibiotics

1 D
2 C
3 A
4 C

2: Perioperative Management 2

1 In wound healing:

A Myofibroblasts appear in the wound at 1 week

B Platelet-derived growth factor is released from arterial smooth muscle cells

C Vitamin A impairs wound healing

D Matrix remodelling occurs at 5–10 days following the formation of a wound

E Excess loss of epithelium often results in healing by primary intention

2 Colonic anastomotic leakage:

A Is confirmed by barium contrast radiography as the investigation of choice

B Is more common than oesophageal anastomotic leakage

C Pyrexia and tachycardia are late features

D Zinc deficiency is a risk factor

E Is more common in the elderly

3 The following have been shown to reduce wound infection:

A Shaving the proposed area of surgery the day before the operation

B Use of single dose prophylactic antibiotics

C Use of interrupted sutures

D Preoperative showering with chlorhexidine

E Use of drains

4 Keloid scars:

A Are characterized by increased lysis of collagen

B May be reduced in size by local steroid injections

C Radiotherapy is a risk factor

D May be reduced in size by Z-plasty

E Typically continue to enlarge for many years

5 Abdominal wound dehiscence:

A Carries a mortality of greater than 20%

B Should not be resutured due to the risk of infection

C Is complicated by incisional hernia in 5% of cases

D Is seldom characterized by a premonitory serous discharge

E Usually occurs during the first and second postoperative days

6 Postoperative pulmonary embolism:

A Chest pain is a characteristic feature

B The pulmonary artery pressure commonly rises

C Chest radiography is typically normal

D Streptokinase may be given

E An ECG may show an S wave in lead II, a Q wave in lead III and T wave in lead III

7 In a 70 kg man:

A The intravascular fluid volume represents 9% of total body weight

B Total extracellular sodium content is approximately 2000 mmol

C Calcium is shared equally between the skeletal and extracellular compartments

D Daily fluid maintenance per unit body weight is lower than for children weighing less than 10 kg

E Sodium and water maintenance requirements are increased in the first 24 to 48 hours postoperatively

8 Fluid and electrolyte maintenance:

A Dextrose saline is the only crystalloid fluid required to replace basal sodium and fluid requirements

B Gelofusine contains dextran 70 as its predominant colloid type

C Ringer's solution contains sodium at a concentration of 30 mmol/L

D 5% dextrose contains 120 kCal/L

E Hartmann's solution contains 29 mmol HCO_3 per litre

9 Regarding the assessment of nutritional state:

A Body Mass Index (BMI) is a reliable indicator of fat and muscle reserve

B Obesity is defined as a BMI greater than 30

C Malnutrition is indicated by a BMI less than 20

D Albumin supplementation is the preferred treatment option for correcting hypoalbuminaemia

E Triceps skinfold thickness may be used to assess muscle mass

10 Feeding:

A By the enteral route promotes blood flow to the gut

B By the enteral route may be complicated by sinusitis

C By the parenteral route (TPN) is only given through central lines

D By TPN may be complicated by lipaemia

E By the enteral route is the first choice method of feeding for trauma patients

11 Blood:

A All black patients need a sickle cell test preoperatively

B Patients with sickle-cell trait are at risk of a crisis in unpressurized aircraft

C HbA represents 95% of the total adult haemoglobin

D The spleen and liver both shrink in size during a sequestration crisis

E Priapism from sickle-cell disease is most appropriately treated conservatively

12 The following are recognized features of anaemia:

A Paronychia

B Shiny tongue

C Angina

D Reduced plasma volume indicating a physiological anaemia

E Dysphagia

13 The following are recognized features of haemophilia A:

A Prolonged prothrombin time

B Thrombocytopenia

C Factor VIII Von Willebrand antigen deficiency

D X-linked dominant inheritance

E Increased factor VIII levels secondary to desmopressin

14 Blood transfusions are routinely screened for:

A Antibodies to HIV-2

B Antibodies to hepatitis B

C Hepatitis C antigen

D Antibodies to *Treponema pallidum*

E Antibodies to cytomegalovirus

15 Absolute indications for the transfusion of fresh frozen plasma include:

A Plasma exchange

B Reversal of the action of warfarin

C Thrombotic thrombocytopenic purpura

D Disseminated intravascular coagulation

E A platelet count below 50×10^9/L before major surgery

16 Complications of massive blood transfusion include:

A Thrombocytopenia

B Air embolism

C Hypokalaemia

D Metabolic alkalosis

E Hypocalcaemia

17 The thrombin time is prolonged in:

A Heparin therapy

B Idiopathic thrombocytopenic purpura

C Liver disease

D Dysfibrinogenaemia

E Von Willebrand's disease

18 Complications of red cell transfusion:

A Non-haemolytic reactions are the most severe

B Urticaria is due to cross reaction to plasma proteins

C Include hyperkalaemia

D Group O rhesus positive blood is the universal donor

E The direct Coombs' test (DCT) detects antibodies on red cells

19 Platelets:
A Are typically stored at –30 °C
B One unit is created from 12–15 donations
C Are stored in a solution containing citrate, phosphate, dextrose and adenine
D May be contaminated with red blood cells
E Require the testing of rhesus compatibility before transfusion

20 Regarding the immune system:
A T lymphocytes survive for under 1 year
B B lymphocytes are commonly situated in the cortex of lymph nodes
C T lymphocytes are characteristically situated in the follicle centres of lymph nodes
D T lymphocytes are more mobile than B lymphocytes
E B lymphocytes make up 60–70% of peripheral lymphocytes

21 Postoperative pyrexia:
A Secondary to a transfusion reaction typically occurs after 250 mL of blood has been given
B Secondary to atelectasis requires the prescription of antibiotics once sputum samples have been sent
C Is unlikely to be caused by a urinary tract infection
D Is rarely caused by thrombophlebitis
E Should be treated with broad-spectrum antibiotics when the cause is unknown

22 Obesity is associated with an increased risk of:
A Perioperative haemorrhage
B Myocardial infarction
C Cerebro-vascular accident
D Anastomotic failure
E Wound dehiscence

23 Protein loss after trauma:
A Nitrogen loss occurs in proportion to the degree of sepsis
B Is greatest in the elderly
C Reaches a peak at 2 weeks
D Occurs principally from liver stores
E Arginine is the major energy source for the gastrointestinal tract

24 After trauma:
A The flow phase is followed by the ebb phase
B The metabolic rate rapidly increases after surgery
C Carbohydrate stores are the main energy source
D Lipolysis occurs secondary to hypoinsulinaemia
E Hyponatraemia results from increased renal losses

25 The typical response to surgery includes:
A An increase in growth hormone
B A decrease in anti-diuretic hormone
C An increase in adrenal corticotrophic hormone
D A decreased urine osmolality
E An increase in glucagon

EXTENDED MATCHING QUESTIONS

Topic: Acid–base balance

A Metabolic acidosis
B Metabolic alkalosis
C Acute respiratory acidosis
D Chronic respiratory acidosis
E Respiratory alkalosis

For each of the results below, select the most likely diagnosis from the list of options above. Each option may be used once, more than once or not at all.

1 pH 7.20 pO_2 94 mmHg
   pCO_2 20 HCO_3 7.0

2 pH 7.25 pO_2 64 mmHg
   pCO_2 58 HCO_3 26

3 pH 7.33 pO_2 70 mmHg
   pCO_2 70 HCO_3 38

4 pH 7.50 pO_2 74 mmHg
   pCO_2 52 HCO_3 34

Topic: Anaemia

A Iron deficiency anaemia
B Sickle-cell anaemia
C Hypothryroidism
D Aplastic anaemia
E Sideroblastic anaemia
F Autoimmune haemolytic anaemia

For each of the results below, select the most likely diagnosis from the list of options above. Each option may be used once, more than once or not at all.

1 Hb 8.4 g/dL   WCC 6.2×10^9/L
   Plt 240×10^9/L   MCV 111 fL

2 Hb 9.2 g/dL   WCC 8.1×10^9/L
   Plt 170×10^9/L   MCV 74 fL

3 Hb 5.4 g/dL   WCC 0.3×10^9/L
   Plt 31×10^9/L   MCV 84 fL

Topic: Hypersensitivity reactions

A Type I
B Type II
C Type III
D Type IV

For each of the disorders below, select the most likely hypersensitivity type from the list of options above. Each option may be used once, more than once or not at all.

1 Systemic lupus erythematosus
2 Contact dermatitis
3 Goodpasture's disease
4 Autoimmune haemolytic anaemia
5 Positive Mantoux Test

ANSWERS TO MULTIPLE CHOICE QUESTIONS

1 In wound healing:
A False
B True
C True
D False
E False

Healing by *primary intention* occurs when wound edges are brought into apposition whereas by *secondary intention* occurs as a result of the formation of granulation tissue in the base of the wound. The cells involved in wound healing include neutrophils which arrive within the first few hours of wound formation, and macrophages whose influx begins within a day or so. Fibroblasts and myofibroblasts enter after 2 or more days and endothelial cells are seen within 5 days. Matrix remodelling occurs *after* 10 days. Platelet derived growth factor (PDGF) is produced by smooth muscle cells. Deficiencies of protein, vitamins A and C and zinc result in impaired wound healing.

2 Colonic anastomotic leakage:
A False
B False
C False
D True
E True

A gastrograffin water soluble contrast study is the preferred investigation of choice for a suspected colonic anastomotic leakage rather than barium as the latter may be complicated by severe peritonitis. Oesophageal leaks are considerably more common than colonic leaks. **Predisposing factors** are similar to those of poor wound healing and can be divided into *general patient related factors* (the elderly, malnutrition, zinc and vitamin C deficiency, diabetes, renal failure, hepatic disease), *local factors* (malignancy and poor blood supply), and *poor surgical technique*. Pyrexia and tachycardia are early clinical features at which stage the patient will usually still have an ileus.

3 The following have been shown to reduce wound infection:
A False
B True
C False
D False
E False

Shaving more than 12 hours preoperatively markedly increases the wound infection rate, as this may expose new bacteria to the skin surface which can multiply avidly prior to the operation. Shaving at the time of surgery is carried out in part to facilitate the application of dressings, and if not performed will not increase the rate of infection. Antibiotic prophylaxis has been shown to reduce the rate of wound infections significantly, and single dose prophylaxis is adequate for many operations. Good haemostasis is preferable to the insertion of a drain as the latter may increase the likelihood of infection if left *in situ* for a prolonged period of time.

4 Keloid scars:
A False
B True
C False
D False
E False

Keloid scars are characterized by excessive production and contraction of fibrous tissue with an increase in collagen synthesis. **Hypertrophic scars** but not keloid scars are characterized by an increased lysis of collagen. Maximum expansion of hypertrophic scars usually occurs by 6 months, whereas keloid scars may continue to expand with time. Treatment should be delayed for at least 6 months until the scar is fully mature. Hypertrophic scars are rarely treated as they tend to regress with time. Keloid scars may be treated with radiotherapy or with steroid injections such as triamcinolone. Alternatively they may be re-excised when mature together with a Z-plasty or other plastic surgical procedure if required. Z-plasty by itself does not reduce the size of a keloid scar but merely acts to re-orientate an ugly scar thereby making it less noticeable.

5 Abdominal wound dehiscence:

A True
B False
C False
D False
E False

Wound dehiscence occurs in less than 0.1% of abdominal operations and represents a disruption of all layers of the abdominal wall. The risk factors which affect dehiscence are numerous and include *general factors* such as coexisting medical illnesses, obesity, malnutrition, malignancy, steroids; *local factors* including infection, ischaemia, foreign bodies; and *poor surgical technique*. There is often a premonitory serosanguinous discharge usually occurring after the fifth postoperative day. Mortality may be as high as 40% and so prompt treatment is essential. This includes adequate resuscitation and analgesia followed by re-exploration with lavage and re-suturing. Incisional hernia complicates about one-quarter of cases.

6 In postoperative pulmonary embolism:

A False
B False
C True
D True
E False

Postoperative **pulmonary emboli** classically occur on day 7 to 10 following a prolonged period of immobilization. Breathlessness, tachycardia, hypotension, haemoptysis, cyanosis and pleuritic pain are recognized features although chest pain does not occur in the majority of cases. The chest X-ray is often normal but may show an effusion or collapse. The ECG may be normal, may show a sinus tachycardia only, or in rare instances may show the classic picture of an S wave in lead I, a Q wave in lead III and a T wave in lead III. Clinical diagnosis is usually confirmed by ventilation–perfusion (V/Q) scanning, and spiral CT may be useful in difficult cases. Signs of deep venous thrombosis should be sought. The pulmonary artery pressure may rise but this only occurs with large central emboli. Pulmonary angiography may occasionally be indicated with a view to either thrombolytic therapy with streptokinase, or more rarely surgical intervention in cases of massive emboli.

7 In a 70 kg man:

A True
B True
C False
D True
E False

In a 70 kg man, total body water approximates to 42 litres (i.e. two-thirds of total body weight) of which extracellular fluid represents 14 L and intracellular fluid 28 L. Total blood volume equates to 5 L, of which 3.5 L is plasma (part of the extracellular compartment) and 1.5 L is cells (from the intracellular compartment). The sodium concentration in extracellular fluid is approximately 140 mmol/L, giving a total sodium content of 1960 mmol. Daily fluid maintenance for children less than 10 kg in weight is 100 mL/kg or 4 mL/kg/hour, compared to 40 mL/kg or 1–2 mL/kg/hour in adults. For the first 1 to 2 days after an operation there is a tendency towards water retention, and sodium retention may continue for several days. Potassium continues to be lost via renal excretion during this period but parenteral supplementation should only be given if the patient has a good urine output. The skeleton contains 99% of the body's calcium, with the extracellular compartment containing a total of 22.5 mmol.

8 Fluid and electrolyte maintenance:

A True
B False
C False

D False
E True

A total of 2.5 litres of dextrose saline will provide the daily basal water and sodium requirements for a 70 kg man. Gelofusine contains succinylated gelatin as its colloid. Dextran 70 is an example of a different type of colloid based on the glucose polymer. It is a good plasma substitute but has adverse effects on coagulation and cross-matching. Ringer's solution or Hartmann's contains 131 mmol Na^+, 5 mmol K^+ and 29 mmol HCO_3^- (as lactate) per litre and with an osmolarity of 280 mOsm/L. Five per cent dextrose contains about 220 kCal/L and therefore on its own will not meet the body's energy requirements.

9 **Regarding the assessment of nutritional state:**
A True
B False
C True
D False
E False

Body Mass Index is calculated by dividing the patient's weight in kilograms by the square of their height in metres. It is a reliable indicator of body size. Normal BMI is 20–25 kg/m²; obesity is classified as a BMI between 25 and 30 and morbid obesity as a BMI in excess of 30. Malnutrition is a BMI <20, with severe malnutrition <16. *Mid-arm circumference* is used as an indicator of muscle mass whereas *triceps skinfold thickness* is an index of fat. *Hypoalbuminaemia* is almost always a manifestation of underlying disease; the priority must therefore be towards treating the primary cause as albumin supplementation on its own will only increase the plasma albumin level temporarily.

10 **Feeding:**
A True
B True
C False
D True
E True

Enteral nutrition has several beneficial effects if given early to trauma patients. Its principle advantage is that it promotes blood flow to the gut thereby reducing the translocation of bacterial endotoxins. It is a cheap and safe method of feeding although there are complications with its use, such as those associated with malposition of the feeding tube, sinusitis or diarrhoea. Total parenteral nutrition (TPN) can be given through a central line or via a PIC line which is a peripheral long line fed centrally. The use of glyceryl trinitrate patches on peripheral cannula sites may prolong their usage. There are many complications associated with TPN including lipaemia, hyperglycaemia, electrolyte abnormalities and abnormal liver function tests.

11 **Blood:**
A True
B True
C True
D False
E False

Sickle-cell anaemia results in severe haemolysis in homozygotes, and may adversely affect heterozygotes in situations of hypoxia, such as in unpressurized aircraft or when subject to anaesthetics. All black people require a sickle screen preoperatively, for example using the *sickledex* test. Priapism lasting longer than 24 hours requires cavernosus-spongiosum shunting if simple aspiration of corpora cavernosum blood proves to be ineffective. Both the spleen and liver enlarge during a sequestration crisis due to trapping of red blood cells. Adult haemoglobin comprises 95% HbA and a small amount of HbA_2. HbF mainly occurs in fetal life or β-thalassaemia.

12 **The following are recognized features of anaemia:**
A True
B True
C True
D False
E True

Anaemia is defined as a reduction in the haemoglobin level below the normal range after correction for the individual's age and sex. In practice this means an Hb below 13.5 g/dL in men and below 11.5 g/dL in women. Koilonychia, stomatitis, atrophic glossitis, post-cricoid web and dysphagia support the diagnosis of iron deficiency anaemia. Anaemia in a patient with ischaemic heart disease may precipitate angina. Physiological anaemia characteristically occurs in pregnancy and is due to an increased plasma volume.

13 The following are recognized features of haemophilia A:

A False
B False
C False
D False
E True

Haemophilia A is a sex-linked recessive condition which occurs in one in ten thousand males. It results in a prolonged APTT due to a deficiency of factor VIII. Carriers are detected by the presence of half the normal level of factor VIII and an imbalance in the ratio between factor VIIIc and vWF levels. *Desmopressin* increases factor VIII levels and may be sufficient in the treatment of mild disease. Major bleeding requires factor VIII levels to be raised to 50% of normal, which may necessitate cryoprecipitate or virally inactivated factor VIII. Factor VIII Willebrand factor antigen deficiency is Von Willebrand's disease, which is an autosomal dominant deficiency of factor VIII related antigen. There is a prolonged bleeding time but a normal platelet count.

14 Blood transfusions are routinely screened for:

A True
B False
C False
D True
E False

Blood in the UK is tested for hepatitis B surface antigen, antibodies to hepatitis C, antibodies to human immunodeficiency virus type 1 and type 2, and *Treponema pallidum* antibodies.

15 Absolute indications for the transfusion of fresh frozen plasma include:

A False
B True
C True
D True
E False

Fresh frozen plasma (FFP) is available in units of 150–300 mL and is stored at –30 °C. It contains all the clotting factors and must be used within an hour of defrosting. Due to red blood cell contamination it is usually given in an ABO compatible form. FFP can be stored for up to one year, unlike red cells which can only be stored for 35 days, and platelets for only 5 days. The *absolute indications* include warfarin reversal, disseminated intravascular coagulation, and thrombotic thrombocytopenic purpura. *Relative indications* include bleeding or disturbed coagulation associated with massive transfusion, liver disease and cardiopulmonary bypass surgery. It can also be used when individual clotting factors are unavailable. Cryoprecipitate may also be given in cases where the fibrinogen concentration is below 1.0 g/L.

16 Complications of massive blood transfusion include:

A True
B True
C False
D True
E True

Massive transfusion is by definition the replacement of total blood volume within a 24 hour period. Complications include hyperkalaemia, hypocalcaemia, metabolic alkalosis, hypothermia, thrombocytopenia, coagulation abnormalities and disseminated intravascular coagulation. Air embolism is a recognized complication if the transfusion is set up incorrectly.

17 The thrombin time is prolonged in:
A True
B False
C True
D True
E False

Idiopathic thrombocytopenic purpura will cause a fall in the platelet count. Heparin therapy, fibrinogen deficiency and liver disease may result in a prolonged thrombin time, as well as an increase in the PT and APTT. Von Willebrand's disease will result in a prolonged APTT.

18 Complications of red cell transfusion:
A False
B True
C True
D False
E True

Acute haemolytic reactions are the most severe of the transfusion reactions. Only a small amount of blood is required to result in shock, disseminated intravascular coagulation (DIC) and renal failure. **Non-haemolytic pyrexia** may follow transfusion and is a result of the formation of antibodies to white blood cells. **Urticarial reactions** are due to plasma proteins including IgA. **Anaphylaxis** may also occur, occasionally as a reaction to plasma proteins in the transfusion. The **delayed haemolytic reaction** is characterized by haemolysis which typically occurs one week after transfusion, and is due to red cell alloantibodies.

Group O is the universal donor of cell transfusions. Rhesus negative blood should be given to women of child-bearing age although rhesus positive blood is advised for older women in the interests of preserving stocks of the universal donor. The direct Coombs' test (DCT) detects antibodies on red cells and is also useful in the diagnosis of haemolytic anaemias.

19 Platelets:
A False
B False
C False
D True
E True

Platelets are stored at about 20 °C and must be used within 5 days. Each unit of 300 mL is drawn from a pool of between 4 and 6 donations and is suspended in plasma. It is important that platelets are given as ABO and Rhesus D compatible units.

20 Regarding the immune system:
A False
B True
C False
D True
E False

T lymphocytes comprise 60–70% of peripheral lymphocytes and are present in the blood, paracortical area of lymph nodes and periarteriolar sheaths in the spleen. They survive for 5 to 10 years. **B lymphocytes** make up 20–30% of peripheral lymphocytes and are found in the bone marrow, lymphoid tissues, and extra-lymphatic organs. In the lymph node they reside in the cortex. They survive for under one year. B lymphocytes form plasma cells which produce immunoglobulins of which 95% are of the IgG, IgM and IgA types. T lymphocytes are more mobile than B lymphocytes.

21 Postoperative pyrexia:
A False
B False
C False
D False
E False

Transfusion reactions can occur after only a small amount of blood has been transfused, and five millilitres may be enough to cause an acute haemolytic reaction. Postoperative atelectasis is common, does not necessarily imply the presence of infection, and therefore does not routinely require the administration of antibiotics. Sputum samples should be sent off, and the patient encouraged to take deep breaths and be assessed by the physiotherapist. Urinary tract infection may present as postoperative pyrexia as well as causing other symptoms. Thrombophlebitis is a frequently missed but surprisingly common cause of postoperative pyrexia particularly with multiple sites of intravenous access, typically occurring 2 weeks following surgery. In postoperative pyrexia, antibiotics should only be used when an infective source is detected and then only once appropriate blood and urine samples and swabs have been sent to microbiology.

22 Obesity is associated with an increased risk of:

A True
B True
C True
D True
E True

Obesity is associated with a number of medical conditions including ischaemic heart disease, diabetes and hypertension. Obese patients, especially those who are morbidly obese are at an increased risk of haematoma formation, infection, dehiscence, anastomotic failure, incisional hernias as well as myocardial infarction and cerebro-vascular accident. Respiratory complications are also more common with an increased incidence of atelectasis. Immobility also results in an increased rate of deep vein thrombosis. It may also be more difficult to make an accurate clinical diagnosis in the presence of obesity.

23 Protein loss after trauma:

A True
B False
C False
D True
E False

Nitrogen loss occurs in proportion to the degree of trauma, sepsis and muscle bulk, being greater in young muscular men and less in the elderly. Loss of amino acids is greatest at *one week* resulting in gluconeogenesis, oxidation of amino acids in the tissues and the formation of acute phase reactants. *Glutamine* is the major energy source for the gastrointestinal tract.

24 After trauma:

A False
B False
C False
D True
E False

Following trauma, the '*ebb*' phase is characterized by an immediate decrease in metabolic rate. When the metabolic rate starts to increase, this phase is followed by the '*flow*' phase. Glycogen stores last for 24 hours before gluconeogenesis occurs in which muscle is broken down to release amino acids. The hyperglycaemia that follows trauma is partly maintained by insulin resistance or 'diabetes of injury'. This is despite insulin levels actually increasing during the flow phase. One of the consequences of the relative insulin resistance is lipolysis resulting in the production of ketones and fatty acids which contribute to the provision of further energy. Water retention due to reduced water clearance occurs within the first 24 hours of trauma and is followed by sodium retention. These effects occur secondary to the release of aldosterone and antidiuretic hormone (ADH). Thus in the very early postoperative period there is a tendency towards a positive fluid balance which necessitates careful fluid management. Too much fluid may result in metabolic alkalosis which itself impairs oxygen delivery to tissues by shifting the oxygen dissociation curve to the left.

25 The typical response to surgery includes:

A True
B False
C True
D False
E True

Perioperatively there is an increase in the concentration of a number of hormones. These are triggered by different stimuli such as *pain* which causes release of anti-diuretic hormone (ADH), aldosterone and catecholamines, *tissue damage* resulting in cytokine release, *infection* resulting in endotoxinaemia, *hypovolaemia* causing sympathetic overdrive and the stimulation of the renin-angiotensin-aldosterone axis, and *relative starvation*. These stimuli are in addition to changes occurring to other parameters such as hypoxia, hypercarbia, hypoglycaemia and hypothermia. The release of ADH and aldosterone result in water retention and an increase in urine osmolality. Diuresis is a good sign of recovery after trauma. Increased levels of adrenal corticotrophic hormone (ACTH) and glucagon also occur and have influences leading to an increase in growth hormone. Other factors stimulating the production of growth hormone include thyroxine, hypovolaemia, hypoglycaemia and the amino acid arginine. The effects of growth hormone are an increased protein synthesis, reduced carbohydrate and fat, and insulin resistance leading to hyperglycaemia.

ANSWERS TO EXTENDED MATCHING QUESTIONS

Topic: Acid–base balance

1 A
The pH is low whilst the pCO_2 is within the normal range indicating an acidosis of metabolic origin.

2 C
This is an acute rather than chronic respiratory acidosis because the pH is still low and has not yet been compensated for by a metabolic alkalosis.

3 D
In this case the pH is nearly within the normal range, and the bicarbonate has increased to above normal levels indicating the development of a compensatory metabolic alkalosis due to renal excretion of H^+ and reabsorption of HCO_3^-.

4 B
The raised pH indicates an alkalosis which is metabolic as the pCO_2 is not raised.

Topic: Anaemia

1 C
This macrocytic (high MCV) anaemia is a feature of hypothyroidism.

2 A
This is a microcytic (low MCV) anaemia typical of iron deficiency.

3 D
In this case the haemoglobin, white cell count and platelet count are all markedly reduced.

Topic: Hypersensitivity reactions

1 C
This occurs by immune complex deposition.

2 A
This results from IgE mediated degranulation of mast cells resulting in the release of various inflammatory agents.

3 B
This is via antibody–antigen binding.

4 B

5 D
This is delayed type or cell mediated hypersensitivity typical of mycobacterium infection.

3: Trauma

MULTIPLE CHOICE QUESTIONS

1 In the management of a multiply injured patient:

A The casualty must be rolled onto his back to assess the airway

B Breathing should be assessed alongside cervical spine control

C Abdominal CT is a useful investigation in the assessment of a shocked patient with intra-abdominal bleeding

D Morphine may mask the presentation of an intracranial bleed

E Jaw thrust is contraindicated in the presence of cervical spine injury

2 In a multiply injured patient, diagnostic peritoneal lavage:

A Should be carried out in the presence of extraluminal air

B Is positive in the presence of more than 100 000 red blood cells per mm^3

C Is contraindicated in the presence of pelvic fractures

D Is indicated in the presence of hypotension of unknown cause

E Is 75% sensitive for intra-abdominal bleeding

3 Indications for thoracotomy in a multiply injured patient include:

A An initial haemothorax of 1200 mL

B An open pneumothorax

C Persistent drainage of 400 mL of blood from a chest drain over 4 hours

D A laceration of the left hemidiaphragm

E Flail chest

4 Features of aortic rupture typically include:

A Fractured third and fourth ribs

B Widened mediastinum

C An upward shift of the left mainstem bronchus

D CT as the investigation of choice

E Penetrating rather than blunt injuries as the cause

5 The following are true about intraosseous infusion:

A It is indicated for children under the age of ten

B Access can be obtained via the tibia in the presence of a tibial fracture on the same side

C Access can be obtained via the distal femur

D Bicarbonate infusions may not be given by this route

E May be complicated by physeal plate injuries

6 In cervical spine injuries:

A Clearance of spinal injuries may be deferred in the presence of adequate immobilization

B Flaccid arreflexia is a feature

C The ability to extend but not flex the elbow supports the diagnosis

D Rupture of the anterior longitudinal ligament is characteristically stable

E A teardrop injury is unstable

7 Cranial nerves:

A Some of the spinal accessory nerve fibres contribute to the pharyngeal plexus

B Abducent nerve lesions correlate poorly with the position of the compressive lesion

C In oculomotor nerve lesions, the eye turns down and in

D A lesion of the left second cranial nerve

at the level of the optic tract causes a right homonymous hemianopia with macular sparing

E Injury to the 12th cranial nerve causes the tongue to deviate to the side of the lesion

8 Indications for a CT in a head injury patient include:

A Post-traumatic seizures

B A progressive deterioration in neurological status

C A skull fracture on X-ray

D A Glasgow Coma Score of 10 on admission

E A young patient with non-progressive headache and vomiting after head injury

9 Immobilization of the cervical spine:

A Is carried out by means of sandbags, soft collar and tape in all patients involved in road traffic accidents

B Should only be discontinued after an orthopaedic assessment

C Should be followed by radiography in all patients

D Normal radiographs exclude a cervical spine injury

E Should ideally be carried out in the position in which the patient is found

10 Regarding blast injuries:

A A shock wave is a low pressure waveform formed by conversion of explosives into gaseous products at high temperature

B Shock waves have a bigger amplitude than sound waves

C Primary effects are caused by missiles accelerated by blast winds

D Traumatic amputation typically occurs as a secondary effect

E Blast lung syndrome commonly occurs amongst survivors

11 Skin loss and donation:

A Allografts are skin transfers in the same patient

B Xenografts are skin transfers between different patients

C A free flap involves a vascular pedicle

D A split skin graft takes 48–72 hours to establish a blood supply

E Split skin grafts cannot usually be recropped within 4 weeks of initial harvesting

12 After a head injury:

A The patient must be intubated and ventilated

B Hyperventilation may result in an increase in intracranial pressure

C An increase in blood pressure directly leads to an increase in intracranial pressure

D Mannitol and steroids should be given to patients with raised intracranial pressure

E Patients should be fitted with a soft collar in case of neck muscle spasm

13 Tension pneumothorax:

A Should be confirmed by a chest radiograph

B Causes mediastinal shift towards, and tracheal shift away from, the abnormal side

C Is treated by a chest drain in the second intercostal space, mid-clavicular line

D Is most commonly caused by penetrating injuries

E May result in cardiac arrest typically due to ventricular fibrillation

14 Regarding the mandible:

A A fracture at the neck results in the medial pterygoid muscle displacing the condyle forwards and medially

B A fracture at the angle results in the ramus being displaced upwards, forwards and medially

C Fractures of this bone form part of the Le Fort III classification

D Bilateral fractures of the body may result in anterior displacement of the central segment

E Airway impairment may occur with bilateral fractures of the body

15 **Features of cardiac tamponade typically include:**

A Distended neck veins
B Pulsus alternans
C Increased blood pressure
D Reduced heart sounds
E Treatment by needle thoracocentesis through the left fifth intercostal space, mid-clavicular line

16 **Features of acute blood loss of 1700 mL in a 70 kg man include:**

A Coma
B A urinary output of 15–20 mL/hour
C A respiratory rate of greater than 40/min
D A pulse rate of 120–140 beats per minute
E A rise in pulse pressure

17 **Burn injuries:**

A Full thickness burns are characteristically less painful than those of partial thickness
B Alkali burns are more damaging than those due to acid
C Full thickness burns amounting to greater than 30% body area should be referred to a designated burns unit
D Should be irrigated with copious amounts of cold running water
E Result in hypothermia when the body temperature falls below 32 °C

18 **Le Fort II maxillofacial fractures:**

A Are commonly associated with basal skull fractures
B Usually involve the pterygoid plates
C May give rise to otorrhoea
D Extend from the nasal bones into the medial orbital wall and cross the infraorbital rim
E Must be managed with consideration given to protection of the airway

19 **The following pairings of radiological features and possible diagnoses are correct:**

A Nasogastric tube in thoracic cavity — Ruptured oesophagus
B Sternal fracture — Cervical spine injury
C Fractured ribs 3–5 — Great vessel injury
D Lumbar spine fracture — Pancreatic injury
E Pubic diastasis — Urethral injury

20 **Regarding high lesions of the brachial plexus:**

A Claw hand is a characteristic sign
B Klumpke's palsy is a rare birth injury
C Hyperextension of the metacarpophalangeal joints may be a feature
D Internal rotation of the arm typically occurs
E Loss of sensation in the ulna distribution of the hand is commonly seen

21 **Regarding median nerve palsy:**

A High lesions may follow elbow dislocation
B Loss of sensation over the medial aspect of the hand is characteristic
C A positive Froment's sign is pathognomonic
D Lesions of the anterior interosseus branch usually result in sensory loss
E Adductor pollicis paralysis typically occurs in low lesions

22 **Nerve injuries affecting the lower limb:**

A A lesion of the L3 or L4 nerve root will result in weakness of knee flexion
B A lesion of the S1 root will result in loss of the ankle reflex
C Sensory loss on the dorsum of the foot characteristically follows an injury to the common peroneal nerve
D Femoral nerve lesions usually result in weak knee extension
E Eversion but not dorsiflexion of the foot is possible following a superficial peroneal nerve lesion

23 **Compartment syndrome:**

A Is usually painful
B Does not present in the upper limbs
C Diagnosis characteristically involves the absence of distal pulses
D Compartment pressures greater than 10 mmHg support the diagnosis
E Fasciotomy should always be done

24 Paediatric trauma:

A Rib fractures are more likely in younger patients than in adults

B Nasotracheal intubation is safer in children than adults

C An infant with a pulse of 160 bpm, systolic BP of 80 mmHg, and a respiratory rate of 40 per minute is in type II shock

D A loss in blood volume of 5–10% is required to produce clinical evidence of shock

E A fluid challenge of 20 mL/kg of crystalloid is typically used

25 Regarding fat embolism:

A Very low density lipoproteins are usually implicated

B Petechial haemorrhages are characteristic

C It is more common in multiple closed than open fractures

D Respiratory alkalosis typically occurs

E Bilateral pleural effusions are a characteristic feature

EXTENDED MATCHING QUESTIONS

Topic: Head injury

A Subarachnoid haemorrhage
B Subdural haematoma
C Extradural haematoma
D Alzheimer's disease
E Multi-infarct dementia

For each clinical presentation, select the most likely diagnosis from the list of options above. Each option may be used once, more than once or not at all.

1 An 83-year-old woman found on the floor at home is diagnosed with a fractured right neck of femur. She becomes increasingly confused on the orthopaedic ward over the next 24 to 48 hours after admission.
2 A 56-year old-man assaulted with a baseball bat with loss of consciousness presents to casualty the same day with a skull fracture on X-ray.
3 A 70-year-old woman with signs of acute progressive dementia over a few weeks' duration.

Topic: Life-threatening injuries

A Cardiogenic shock
B Neurogenic shock
C Septic shock
D Cardiac tamponade
E Tension pneumothorax

For each clinical scenario, select the most likely diagnosis from the list of options above. Each option may be used once, more than once or not at all.

1 Hypotension and bradycardia
2 Hypotension and raised JVP
3 Kussmaul's sign
4 Hypotension and warm peripheries

Topic: Emergency procedures

A Chest X-ray
B Chest drain
C Needle thoracocentesis
D CT abdomen
E Laparotomy
F Cervical spine X-rays
G Diagnostic peritoneal lavage
H Intravenous cannulation

For each clinical scenario, select the most appropriate procedure from the list of options above. Each option may be used once, more than once or not at all.

1 A 19-year-old man involved in a road traffic accident with no obvious external injury presents with a stable airway and cervical spine immobilized. Primary X-rays have been taken. Respiratory rate 22/minute, pulse 110 beats per minute, BP 90 systolic.
2 A 27-year-old woman involved in a road traffic accident presents with an immobilized cervical spine and increased resonance to the left side of her chest.
3 A 21-year-old woman suffers blunt trauma in a head-on collision. Cervical spine immobilized, airway and breathing assessed and stable. Cervical spine X-rays have been taken. Pulse 120 beats per minute, BP 80/50 and normal abdominal appearance.

ANSWERS TO MULTIPLE CHOICE QUESTIONS

1 In the management of a multiply injured patient:

A False
B False
C False
D True
E False

The **Primary Survey** consists of Airway assessment and maintenance with cervical spine control, Breathing and ventilation, Circulation with haemorrhage control, Disability with assessment of neurological status and Exposure/Environmental control.

This sequence provides a priority for assessment and management. CT examination of the abdomen should only be considered in fully stabilized patients. Opiates may result in pupillary constriction and also respiratory depression, and may make diagnosis of intracranial bleeds difficult.

Jaw thrust is a technique used to maintain an airway which avoids hyperextension of the cervical spine and is therefore useful in trauma victims.

2 In a multiply injured patient, diagnostic peritoneal lavage:

A False
B True
C False
D True
E False

Diagnostic peritoneal lavage (DPL) is considered 98% sensitive for intra-abdominal bleeding and is indicated in the evaluation of the hypotensive patient. It is contraindicated in the presence of an absolute indication for laparotomy which includes extraluminal air, gunshot and stab wounds, peritonitis, persistent hypotension, injured diaphragm, perforated bladder and organ injury. *Relative* contra-indications to DPL include obesity, previous abdominal operations, coagulopathy and advanced cirrhosis. In the presence of pelvic fractures, peritoneal lavage should be performed above the umbilicus, and free flow of blood is a positive indication for laparotomy. However, a positive test as determined by the presence of more than 100 000 red blood cells per mm^3 may be false in 15% due to leakage from a retroperitoneal haematoma.

3 Indications for thoracotomy in a multiply injured patient include:

A False
B False
C False
D True
E False

An **emergency thoracotomy** is indicated *immediately* in patients with exsanguinating and penetrating precordial lesions who have no pulse but who have myocardial electrical activity (i.e. electromechanical dissociation, EMD). Blunt injuries rarely require immediate thoracotomy. Indications for thoracotomy as part of the *secondary survey* include patients who have an initial haemothorax of at least 1500 mL or continuing drainage of blood of at least 200 mL per hour for 4 hours, cardiac tamponade, persistent air leak or diaphragmatic lacerations. Flail chest associated with multiple rib fractures is treated with ventilation, humidified oxygen and fluid resuscitation. Traumatic diaphragmatic rupture is treated by direct repair and may follow both blunt and penetrating trauma. A pneumothorax is best treated by chest drain insertion with connection to an underwater seal apparatus.

4 Features of aortic rupture typically include:

A False
B True
C False
D False
E False

Traumatic aortic rupture most commonly results from blunt trauma and is fatal. Aortography is preferred to CT as the investigation of choice for accurate diagnosis. However, chest radiography is a useful first line investigation and its radiographic features may include widened mediastinum, fractures of the first and second ribs, obliteration of the aortic knob, tracheal deviation to the right, pleural cap, elevation of the right and depression of the left mainstem bronchi, deviation of the oesophagus to the right and obliteration of the space between the pulmonary artery and aorta.

5　The following are true about intraosseous infusion:

A　False
B　True
C　True
D　False
E　True

Intraosseous infusion is limited to children 6 years of age and under. It is most commonly performed via the proximal tibial route being inserted 1–3 cm below the tibial tuberosity. Complications include cellulitis, osteomyelitis, fluid extravasation, pressure necrosis, physeal plate injury and haematoma. If the tibia is fractured, the distal femur is an alternative site of access. Infusion can occur proximal but never distal to a fracture site. Intraosseous infusion is for emergency resuscitation and is used when attempted venous access has failed or is impossible due to circulatory collapse. It should be discontinued as soon as adequate venous access is secured.

6　In cervical spine injuries:

A　True
B　True
C　False
D　False
E　True

A lateral cervical spine radiograph should be carried out after life-threatening injuries have been assessed and controlled. This necessitates good immobilization if clearance of the cervical spine is to be deferred. Flaccid arreflexia and the ability to flex but not extend at the elbow are features suggesting cervical spine injury. The anterior longitudinal ligament is part of the first column of stability and if ruptured the injury is usually unstable. Teardrop injuries may be represented as a bony chip from the anteroinferior aspect of the vertebral body and may also indicate posterior displacement of the disc or of a posterior fragment of the vertebral body into the spinal cord.

7　Cranial nerves:

A　False
B　True
C　False
D　False
E　True

The spinal root of the accessory nerve arises from the anterior horn of the upper five cervical cord segments and ascends behind the denticulate ligament to enter the intracranial cavity through the foramen magnum, before joining with the cranial root which arises from the nucleus ambiguus. The combined nerve exits the skull in the jugular foramen. All of the *cranial* fibres join the vagus nerve to contribute to the pharyngeal plexus, whereas the remaining *spinal* root passes into the posterior triangle of the neck to supply sternocleidomastoid and trapezius.

The abducent (sixth) cranial nerve has a long intracranial course, therefore compression by tumours or aneurysms does not reliably indicate their precise anatomical location.

A lesion to the oculomotor (third) cranial nerve causes the eye to look down and out due to unopposed action of the lateral rectus and superior oblique muscles supplied by the abducent and trochlear nerves respectively. There is also ptosis and there *may* be pupillary dilation if the parasympathetic fibres (which travel on the surface of the nerve) are also interrupted, such as by external compression. The pupil does not react to light or accommodation.

A lesion to the **left optic tract** will give rise to a right homonymous hemianopia *without* macular sparing as the latter is a feature of visual cortex lesions where the most posterior part is spared from damage on account of its blood supply arising from a different source (middle cerebral artery).

Injury to the **hypoglossal (twelfth) cranial nerve** results in the tongue deviating to the side of the lesion.

8 Indications for a CT in a head injury patient include:

A   True
B   True
C   False
D   False
E   False

A CT scan is indicated immediately in patients with a GCS ≤ 8 and urgently in patients with unequal pupils, a lateralized defect or an open injury. A fall in GCS or deterioration of neurological status may indicate a worsening intracranial injury and is an emergency. Patients with skull fractures should be admitted for observation. A CT scan is indicated if the fracture is depressed together and neurosurgical advice should be sought. Seizures are common, can occur with any head injury, and may require no treatment. Prolonged seizures may be associated with intracranial haemorrhage and are treated aggressively. Headache and vomiting which are non-progressive are common after a head injury. Patients discharged after minor head injuries should be advised to return if they experience worsening headache, vomiting or other neurological symptoms, and should always be discharged into the care of friends or family.

9 Immobilization of the cervical spine:

A   False
B   False
C   False
D   False
E   False

Any patient with an injury *above the clavicle* or a head injury *resulting in unconsciousness* should be suspected of having an associated cervical spinal injury. Sandbags, *hard* collar and tape must all be used for adequate immobilization of the cervical spine. The neck is immobilized manually in the in-line position without traction. Lateral c-spine radiography is not indicated in all patients arriving with a collar. Each case must be assessed clinically and a lateral c-spine radiograph requested only for those suspected of having a cervical spine injury. This is usually included as one of the three essential radiographs requested as part of the primary survey. The base of the skull, T1 and C7 *must* be visualized. Portable films may miss up to 15% of injuries. A CT scan should be carried out in those cases with a high index of suspicion and negative radiographs.

10 Regarding blast injuries:

A   False
B   True
C   False
D   False
E   False

Shock waves occur on detonation of explosives to form gaseous products at high temperature. They are of high pressure, high velocity and are of a bigger amplitude compared to **sound waves**. *Primary* effects arise from the shock wave itself and cause damage to air-fluid surfaces. *Secondary* effects are caused by the missiles and blast winds, and *tertiary* effects result from total body displacement causing crush injuries and amputations. Blast lung commonly results in death and occurs in confined areas.

11 Skin loss and donation:

A   True
B   True
C   True
D   False
E   False

Grafts are skin transfers from one site to another in which the skin must re-establish its blood supply through numerous dermal and sub-dermal collaterals. In contrast, flaps carry a specified vascular pedicle which is transferred with the skin. *Autografts* occur within the same animal, *allografts* within the same species and *xenografts* between different species. Split-skin grafts take about 24–48 hours to establish a new blood supply and the graft site can usually be recropped after 2 weeks.

12 After a head injury:
A False
B False
C False
D False
E False

Patients with head injuries resulting in unconsciousness must be assumed to have a cervical spine injury and should therefore have full neck immobilization as described above. Management of such a patient follows the sequence ABCDE and intubation with ventilation may be required. Early ventilation should be considered in such patients. Hyperventilation to reduce the $PaCO_2$ to between 26–28 mmHg will reduce the intracranial blood volume by a reduction of cerebrovasodilatation, thereby reducing intracranial pressure. Hyperventilation will also reduce acidosis and increase cerebral metabolism. Cerebral perfusion pressure is the systemic arterial pressure minus the intracranial pressure. As a compensatory mechanism cerebrospinal fluid and/or venous blood can be removed from the intracranial compartment at a faster rate than normal. This can take place up to the equivalent of approximately 50–100 mL of intracranial mass thereby helping to avoid a rise in intracranial pressure. Mannitol may be useful in lowering intracranial pressure and can be used as a delaying tactic rather than a treatment, such as prior to a patient being transferred to a neurosurgical unit. Steroids are not recommended in acute head injury.

13 Tension pneumothorax:
A False
B False
C False
D False
E False

A **tension pneumothorax** is an emergency which results from air being forced into the thoracic cavity and is associated with collapse of the ipsilateral lung and shift of the trachea and mediastinum to the opposite side. It is commonly caused by mechanical ventilation, positive end expiratory pressure (PEEP), blunt trauma or it may be spontaneous due to a ruptured bulla. Treatment is initially by needle decompression in the second intercostal space in the mid-clavicular line, followed by chest drain insertion into the fourth or fifth intercostal space anterior to the mid-axillary line which is carried out at a later stage. Tension pneumothorax is a recognized cause of *electromechanical dissociation (EMD)*. Clinical treatment should NEVER be delayed for radiological investigations due to the urgent nature of the condition.

14 Regarding the mandible:
A False
B True
C False
D False
E True

A fracture at the neck of the mandible results in the *lateral* pterygoid muscle displacing the condyle forwards and medially. A fracture at the angle results in the ramus being displaced upwards, forwards and medially and bilateral fractures of the body may result in posterior displacement of the central part which may lead to airway obstruction. Le Fort III describes the detachment of the middle third of the facial skeleton from the cranial base. It is commonly associated with basal skull fractures and includes fractures to the maxilla, nasal and lacrimal bones, ethmoid, sphenoid, and zygomatic process of the temporal bone.

15 Features of cardiac tamponade typically include:

A True
B False
C False
D True
E False

Only a small amount of blood or fluid is needed to result in cardiac tamponade by mechanically restricting cardiac contraction. It may be characterized by *Beck's triad* which includes a rise in central venous pressure, drop in arterial pressure and muffled heart sounds. Distended neck veins and pulsus paradoxus may be detected. *Kussmaul's sign* is a rise in venous pressure with inspiration and is associated with tamponade.

Pericardiocentesis should be carried out via the sub-xiphoid route aiming the needle towards the tip of the left scapula.

16 Features of acute blood loss of 1700 mL in a 70 kg man include:

A False
B False
C False
D True
E False

Blood loss of this extent is classified as **Class III haemorrhage** and represents 30–40% loss of circulating blood volume. Details of clinical presentation of acute blood loss in a 70 kg man is shown in Table 1.

17 Burn injuries:

A True
B True
C False
D False
E False

Full thickness burns are usually dry and painless compared to **partial thickness burns** which are red and painful. Alkali burns are more serious than acid burns as they tend to be deeper and cause a greater degree of tissue necrosis, thereby requiring longer irrigation. Full and partial thickness burns greater than 10% in a child and 20% in an adult should be referred to a specialist burns unit, particularly if the burn involves the facial and genital areas. Full thickness burns over 5% may require specialist help. Cold running water may cause damage to patients with extensive burns. Hypothermia is defined as a temperature below 35 °C, and is a major risk of extensive burn injuries.

Table 1

70 kg man	Class I	Class II	Class III	Class IV
Blood loss (mL)	<750 (<15%)	750–1500 (15–30%)	1500–2000 (30–40%)	>2000 (>40%)
Pulse rate	<100	>100	>120	>140
Blood pressure	↔	↔	↓	↓
Pulse pressure	↔ / ↑	↓	↓	↓
Respiratory rate	14–20	20–30	30–40	>35
Urine output (mL/hr)	>30	20–30	5–15	negligible
Mental state	anxious	anxious	confusion	confusion, lethargy

18 Le Fort II maxillofacial fractures:

A False
B True
C False
D True
E True

Le Fort II fractures extend from the nasal bones into the medial orbital wall and cross the infraorbital rim. The bones involved include the maxilla, nasal and lacrimal, sphenoid, vomer and ethmoid. Otorrhoea is a feature of basal skull fractures which are commonly associated with Le Fort III fractures. Trauma and fracture of the bones of the maxillofacial skeleton can lead to nerve and blood vessel damage, with the bleeding and deformity resulting in airway compromise.

19 The following pairings of radiological features and possible diagnoses are correct:

A True
B True
C False
D False
E True

Airway or great vessel injury should be suspected in the presence of fractures of the upper three ribs. Pancreatic injury may be associated with lower thoracic spine fractures, and renal injury with lumbar spine fractures. Other trauma-related associations include loss of the psoas shadow and retroperitoneal haematoma, lower rib fractures and hepatic or splenic injury, and sternal fracture and myocardial contusion.

20 Regarding high lesions of the brachial plexus:

A False
B False
C False
D True
E False

High lesions of the brachial plexus involve the C5 and C6 nerve roots and result in paralysis of the abductors and external rotators of the shoulder. The arm hangs close to the body and is internally rotated. Sensation is lost in the lateral aspect of the arm and forearm. When this occurs as a birth injury it is known as *Erb's* palsy, whereas a low lesion at birth is *Klumpke's* palsy. In the latter the intrinsic muscles of the hand are paralyzed and claw-like with hyperextension of the metacarpophalangeal joints and flexion of the interphalangeal joints. Sensation is lost in the ulnar distribution of the hand and forearm.

21 Regarding median nerve palsy:

A True
B False
C False
D False
E False

The **median nerve** is usually injured at the wrist or at a higher level in the forearm. In low lesions there is wasting of the thenar eminence, and thumb abduction and opposition are weak. Sensory loss characteristically occurs over the radial three and one-half digits. High lesions are typically due to forearm fractures or elbow dislocation and in addition to low lesions result in paralysis of the long flexors to the thumb, index and middle fingers. *Froment's* sign indicates an *ulnar* nerve palsy and is due to adductor pollicis weakness. Anterior interosseous nerve lesions result in no sensory loss but cause paralysis of the flexor pollicis longus and of flexor digitorum profundus to the first and second digits.

22 Nerve injuries affecting the lower limb:

A False
B True
C True
D True
E False

Lesions affecting the **L3/4 nerve root** result in weak knee extension and a decreased knee reflex with sensory loss over the anterior thigh and medial part of the leg. **S1** lesions cause weak plantar flexion, loss of the ankle reflex and sensory loss over the sole of the foot. **Common peroneal nerve lesions** may follow pressure from plaster casts and lateral knee ligament injuries. These result in foot drop with weak dorsiflexion and eversion, and sensory loss over the dorsum of the foot and the lateral one-half and anterior aspect of the leg. **Superficial peroneal nerve lesions** impair eversion but not dorsiflexion of the foot as this action is subserved by the deep peroneal nerve.

23 Compartment syndrome:
A True
B False
C False
D False
E True

Muscle swelling due to trauma or ischaemia is contained within its own fascial compartment thereby causing an increase in tissue pressure which ultimately gives rise to compartment syndrome. It may occur in one of the compartments of the leg or forearm, but may involve any space. The pressure required to result in tissue necrosis and therefore necrosis of nerves and muscles is about 40 mmHg. Features include pain worse on passive stretching of the muscles, decreased sensation, tense swelling and weakness of the muscles involved. Limb pulses and capillary filling may be lost as late features. Early fasciotomy is therefore essential.

24 Paediatric trauma:
A False
B False
C False
D False
E True

Rib fractures are uncommon in children due to the pliable nature of their skeleton and when they occur indicate a massive high energy injury. Nasotracheal intubation should be avoided in children due to the relatively acute angle of the nasopharynx. An infant by definition is less than one year of age, and acceptable normal vital signs include a pulse rate of 160 bpm, systolic BP of 80 mmHg and respiratory rate of 40 breaths/min. Approximately one-quarter of the circulating blood volume must be lost before shock is clinically detectable, which should be treated with a fluid challenge of 20 mL/kg. This may be repeated if there is no clinical improvement.

25 Regarding fat embolism:
A False
B True
C True
D True
E False

Fat embolism syndrome typically follows multiple closed long bone fractures but may occur with burns and post-cardiopulmonary bypass. A rise in circulating triglycerides occurs, both due to release from the bone marrow and increased synthesis. Clinical features classically appear 24 to 48 hours after the injury and include mental changes such as confusion, pyrexia, tachycardia, petechial haemorrhages and hypoxaemia associated with acute lung injury (ALI). Pulmonary oedema rather than pleural effusions is the most likely respiratory manifestation. The hyperventilation that results from hypoxaemia leads to a fall in $PaCO_2$ and a respiratory alkalosis.

Topic: Head injury

1 B

It is not uncommon for elderly patients to sustain a head injury as a result of falling to the ground after a hip fracture. This usually manifests itself as a subdural bleed which may be acute or chronic depending on the time period over which it presents.

2 C

Extradural bleeds are associated with a loss of consciousness followed by a lucid period before consciousness deteriorates, contralateral hemiparesis and an ipsilateral fixed and dilated pupil.

3 E

Topic: Life-threatening injuries

1 B
2 A
3 D
4 C

Topic: Emergency procedures

1 H

This is the next procedure which must be carried out in this man. In the absence of assessment and protection of the airway from the list above, it must be assumed that this has already been accomplished alongside control of his cervical spine.

2 C

This is the immediate management of tension pneumothorax but must be followed up by formal chest drain insertion later.

3 G

This lady is haemodynamically compromised. Her chest is unlikely to be the cause from the information given and therefore she has as yet an unexplained source of bleeding. Thus a diagnostic peritoneal lavage is indicated even though the abdomen may *look* normal as long as there is no definite indication for laparotomy.

4: Intensive Care

MULTIPLE CHOICE QUESTIONS

1 Regarding the anterior body wall:
A Venous return from the subcutaneous tissues typically follows the arterial supply
B The thoraco-epigastric vein is a porto-systemic shunt
C Lymphatic drainage of the anterior abdominal wall is to superficial inguinal nodes
D The lateral cutaneous branches of the ilioinguinal and iliohypogastric nerves supply the skin of the buttock
E The breast lymphatics drain to axillary and infraclavicular lymph nodes

2 Causes of mediastinal enlargement include:
A Empyema
B Morgagni hernia
C Hiatus hernia
D Renal cell carcinoma
E Sarcoidosis

3 Structures crossing the neck of the first rib include the:
A Sympathetic trunk
B Subclavian vein
C Subclavian artery
D Superior intercostal artery
E Scalenus anterior muscle

4 The following are features of the adult respiratory distress syndrome:
A Pulmonary artery wedge pressure ≤18 mmHg
B Arterial hypoxaemia which can be reversed by oxygen therapy
C Decreased pulmonary lymph flow
D Thickening of the alveolar capillary membrane

E Abnormalities on the chest X-ray often appear early in the course of the condition

5 The following structures are correctly matched with the vertebral level at which they pass through the diaphragm:
A Thoracic duct — T12
B Oesophagus — T8
C Right vagus nerve — T10
D Right phrenic nerve — T8
E Inferior vena cava — T8

6 Early nutritional support in trauma patients:
A Maintains immune function
B Reduces sepsis
C Has no long term benefit in multiple organ failure
D Increases protein catabolism
E Provides arginine as the main substrate for gut mucosal cells

7 Regarding the bronchi:
A The right main bronchus is shorter than the left
B The left main bronchus gives off no branches before the hilum
C The left pulmonary artery passes inferior to the left main bronchus
D The right bronchial artery is a direct branch of the aorta
E The phrenic nerves lie posterior to the hilum

8 The blood supply to the heart:
A The right coronary artery descends in the atrioventricular groove
B The right coronary artery is larger than the left

C The sinoatrial node is supplied by the left coronary artery in 40% of people
D Has a good collateral supply
E Anterior interventricular artery is more commonly affected by disease than the posterior

9 **Cardiac conduction:**
A The refractory period in cells of the SA and AV nodes is of a shorter duration than in other myocytes
B Purkinje fibres may generate their own rhythm at a rate of 20 beats per minute
C The ST segment is typically isoelectric
D AV node delay is normally 0.25–0.40 s
E The ECG may be entirely normal in the presence of significant cardiac disease

10 **Regarding the cardiovascular system:**
A Tissue perfusion is maximal at normal blood pressures
B Ejection fraction is an index of contractility
C With full autonomic blockade the resting pulse is approximately 70 bpm
D Acidosis increases the sensitivity of myofibrils to calcium
E Digoxin increases the calcium concentration by inhibiting the Na/K/ATPase pump

11 **Cardiac output:**
A Varies directly with central venous pressure over a wide range
B Increases with altitude
C Decreases on standing up
D Decreases with sleep
E May be calculated by oesophageal Doppler

12 **The jugular venous pressure:**
A Increases on standing
B The cannon wave is a large c-wave which may occur in complete heart block
C Is raised in pericardial tamponade
D Increases on inspiration
E Increases with exercise

13 **In the cardiac cycle:**
A The mitral valve opens at the second heart sound
B The c-wave of the JVP occurs at the R wave of the ECG
C Aortic pressure is equal to left ventricular pressure
D Left atrial pressure peaks at the point of closure of the mitral valve
E The third heart sound occurs at the point of opening of the mitral valve

14 **Atrial fibrillation may be associated with:**
A Myocardial infarction
B Hypertension
C Hypothyroidism
D Sarcoidosis
E Carcinoma of the bronchus

15 **Regarding electrocardiographic abnormalities:**
A Hypocalcaemia shortens the Q–T interval
B Hyperkalaemia causes tall T waves and absent P waves
C Right axis deviation may be caused by right bundle branch block
D ST depression may occur in association with a ventricular aneurysm
E Digoxin toxicity causes ST depression and inverted T waves in leads V5 and V6

16 **Complications of acute tubular necrosis include:**
A Hyperkalaemia
B Hypercalcaemia
C Impaired platelet function
D Pericarditis
E Multiple Organ Dysfunction Syndrome

17 **Dopamine:**
A Increases cardiac output
B Increases delivery of diuretic drugs to the distal tubule
C Increases the serum concentration of aldosterone
D Is indicated in oliguric renal failure
E Given at a renal dose has a standard response in most patients

18 In the treatment of pulseless ventricular tachycardia:

A Defibrillation should precede basic life support if available

B 1 mg adrenaline is given every minute

C Synchronized shocks are the preferred method of treatment

D Atropine is not indicated

E May initially look indistinguishable from supraventricular tachycardia on an ECG

19 Causes of hypertension include:

A Polycystic kidneys

B Idiopathic in 70% of cases

C Polyarteritis nodosa

D Hypoparathyroidism

E Acromegaly

20 In a lateral thoracotomy:

A The posterolateral approach is used for transaxillary sympathectomy

B The anterolateral approach is through the sixth rib space

C Latissimus dorsi is divided in the anterolateral approach

D Pectoralis major is divided during oesophageal surgery approached from the left lateral side

E Serratus anterior is spared in the anterolateral approach

21 Regarding arterial lines:

A Hill's test is used to assess the collateral circulation in the hand

B Dorsalis pedis may be used

C Aneurysm formation is a recognized complication

D Arterio-venous fistula is a recognized complication

E Anaemia may result from repeated attempts

22 Complications of tracheostomy include:

A Anoxia

B Air embolism

C Tracheo-oesophageal fistula

D Hypotension

E Tracheal stenosis

23 Causes of hilar enlargement include:

A Sarcoidosis

B Lymphoma

C Hypertension

D Tuberculosis

E Caplan's syndrome

24 Muscles involved in expiration during quiet breathing include:

A Rectus abdominis

B External intercostals

C The diaphragm

D Internal intercostals

E External oblique

25 The following stimulate breathing via the respiratory centre:

A C-fibre receptor stimulation

B Increased pH in the cerebrospinal fluid

C Hypotension

D Muscle spindle receptor stimulation

E Hypercarbia via a direct action on the medullary centre

EXTENDED MATCHING QUESTIONS

Topic: Shock

A Cardiogenic
B Pulmonary oedema
C Septic
D Anaphylactic

For each set of observations, select the most appropriate diagnosis from the list of options above. Each option may be used once, more than once or not at all.

(BP, blood pressure; CO, cardiac output; CVP, central venous pressure)

1	$\downarrow$BP	$\downarrow$CO	$\downarrow$CVP
2	$\downarrow$BP	$\uparrow$CO	$\downarrow$CVP
3	$\downarrow$BP	$\downarrow$CO	$\uparrow$CVP
4	$\rightarrow$BP	$\rightarrow$CO	$\uparrow$CVP

Topic: Respiratory abnormalities

A Tuberculosis
B Fibrosing alveolitis
C Asthma
D Chronic obstructive airways disease
E Simple coal workers' pneumoconiosis

For each set of lung function tests, select the most likely diagnosis from the list of options above. Each option may be used once, more than once or not at all. Normal values are given below each parameter.

	FEV$_1$	FVC	TLC	RV	DLCO	KCO
	2.5–3.5 L	2.3–3.6 L	6.0–8.0 L	2.2–3.0 L	8.0–10.0 L	1.0–1.5 L
1	0.92	2.5	10.6	7.8	3.5	0.5
2	1.3	1.6	3.0	1.0	2.2	1.0

Topic: Nutrition

A Nasogastric tube
B Percutaneous endoscopic gastrostomy
C Surgical gastrostomy
D Needle catheter jejunostomy
E Total parenteral nutrition
F Fluid hydration only

For each patient, select the most appropriate method of early nutrition from the list of options above. Each option may be used once, more than once or not at all.

1 A 52-year-old man undergoing elective right hemicolectomy for adenocarcinoma of the ascending colon.
2 A 63-year-old man undergoing Ivor Lewis operation for oesophageal carcinoma.
3 A 27-year-old woman with multiple injuries on ITU.
4 A 55-year-old man with acute-on-chronic pancreatitis who has extensive tissue necrosis and multiple operative interventions.

1 Regarding the anterior body wall:

A False
B False
C False
D False
E False

The *venous return* from the subcutaneous tissues does not routinely follow the arteries. The blood is collected by an anastomosing network of veins emanating from the umbilicus. Below the umbilicus, blood drains to the great saphenous vein in the groin and above the umbilicus to the lateral thoracic vein. The thoraco-epigastric vein provides a communication between the inferior and superior vena cavae. *Lymphatic drainage* of the abdominal wall above the umbilicus is to axillary nodes, whilst below the umbilicus is to superficial inguinal nodes. Lymphatic drainage of the breast is to axillary and internal thoracic nodes.

The lateral cutaneous branches of T12 and of the iliohypogastrics supply the skin of the buttock. The ilioinguinal nerve is the lateral cutaneous branch of the iliohypogastric nerve, both of which arise from the L1 root. The ilioinguinal nerve itself has no lateral cutaneous branch but has a terminal sensory distribution to the skin of the root of the penis, anterior one-third of the scrotum and a small area below the medial part of the inguinal ligament.

2 Causes of mediastinal enlargement include:

A False
B True
C False
D True
E False

Causes of **mediastinal enlargement** include aortic aneurysm and dissection, lymphadenopathy secondary to lymphoma and metastases, thymoma, retrosternal thyroid, para-oesophageal diverticulum (Zenker's), dermoid cyst, teratoma, bronchogenic cyst, pericardial cyst, Morgagni and Bochdalek diaphragmatic herniae, neurogenic tumours and paravertebral masses.

3 Structures crossing the neck of the first rib include the:

A True
B False
C False
D True
E False

Crossing the neck of the first rib from medial to lateral are the sympathetic trunk, the superior intercostal vein and artery, and the large T1 branch to the brachial plexus. The subclavian artery and vein do not cross the neck of the first rib, but lie posterior and anterior to the scalene tubercle respectively. Scalenus anterior attaches to this tubercle.

4 The following are features of the adult respiratory distress syndrome:

A True
B False
C False
D True
E False

Adult respiratory distress syndrome (ARDS) occurs in cases of Acute Lung Injury (ALI) and has three components: impaired oxygenation, bilateral hilar infiltrates and a pulmonary artery wedge pressure less than or equal to 18 mmHg. It is commonly associated with sepsis and multiple trauma. The release of numerous enzymes and inflammatory mediators cause fluid leakage from capillaries resulting in oedema of the lung tissue. The pulmonary lymph flow is increased and there is thickening of the alveolar-capillary membrane, thereby contributing to a reduction in pulmonary compliance. Arterial hypoxaemia is not corrected by conventional oxygen therapy. The chest radiograph is initially normal but subsequently shows bilateral infiltrates in the lung fields and has a ground glass appearance. These changes are similar to those seen in left ventricular failure or 'cardiogenic' pulmonary oedema, thus these conditions must be excluded by measuring the wedge pressure before a diagnosis of ARDS can be made. Despite treatment with positive end expiratory pressure, permissive hypercapnia and nitric oxide, the mortality is over 50%.

5 The following structures are correctly matched with the vertebral level at which they pass through the diaphragm:
A True
B False
C True
D True
E True

T8
• Inferior vena cava, right phrenic nerve
• Surface marking 1–1.5 cm to the right of the midline at the level of the sixth costal cartilage

T10
• Oesophagus, branches of the left gastric artery and vein, both vagus nerves
• Surface marking 2.5–3 cm to the left of the midline at the level of the seventh costal cartilage

T12
• Aorta, thoracic duct and often the azygos vein
• Surface marking 2.5–3 cm above the transpyloric plane in the midline

Other structures
• Greater, lesser and least splanchnic nerves pierce each crus
• Sympathetic chain passes under the medial arcuate ligament
• Subcostal neurovascular bundle passes under the lateral arcuate ligament
• Left phrenic nerve pierces the left dome of the diaphragm

6 Early nutritional support in trauma patients:
A True
B True
C False
D False
E False

The benefits of **early nutritional support** are well recognized and include a reduction of protein catabolism and infection with maintenance of the immune system. It may also reduce the high mortality associated with multi-organ failure (MOF). *Glutamine* is the main substrate for gut mucosal cells, though *arginine* is an added substrate in enteral feed for its benefits in wound healing and lymphocyte activity.

7 Regarding the bronchi:
A True
B True
C False
D False
E False

The arrangement of structures in the **hilum** of the lung is as follows. The bronchi are centrally placed, with the two pulmonary arteries superior and the pulmonary veins inferior to it. The pulmonary ligament extends in an inferior direction, representing the point at which the visceral and parietal pleura meet. Within the hilum are found lymph nodes, lymphatics, the vagus nerve and sympathetic fibres.

There are *two* bronchial arteries on the *left* which arise directly from the aorta, whereas there is only *one* bronchial artery on the *right* which arises from the right third posterior intercostal artery.

8 The blood supply to the heart:
A True
B False
C True
D False
E True

The **right coronary artery** arises from the anterior aortic sinus and the larger **left coronary artery** from the left posterior aortic sinus. Branches of the right include the conus artery, SA nodal branch (supplying the SA node in 60% of people), marginal branch, AV nodal artery and the posterior interventricular artery. The left coronary artery gives rise to the circumflex and anterior interventricular artery (otherwise known as the left anterior descending artery), the latter being most commonly affected by atheromatous disease. Other branches include a conus branch, diagonal and obtuse marginal branches. The circumflex branch gives origin to the SA nodal artery in 40% of people. There is however considerable variation. There is a poor collateral supply which explains the high incidence of myocardial infarction when an artery occludes.

9 Cardiac conduction:

A True
B False
C True
D False
E True

The cells of the SA node have the highest firing frequency followed by those of the AV node with the Purkinje fibres firing at 30 beats per minute. The AV node delay is represented by the PR interval on the ECG, which is 0.12 to 0.20 seconds. The exercise ECG is a better assessment of ischaemic heart disease than the resting ECG, as the latter may be completely normal even in the presence of significant disease.

10 Regarding the cardiovascular system:

A False
B True
C False
D False
E True

In the presence of a normal blood pressure, peripheral tissue perfusion can be poor if the systemic vascular resistance is raised due to peripheral vasoconstriction. This commonly occurs in the early stages of shock as a mechanism for maintaining a normal blood pressure. Acidosis decreases the sensitivity of myofibrils to calcium. It is therefore negatively inotropic.

The **heart rate** is determined by a balance between the parasympathetic and sympathetic systems. At a normal heart rate of 70 bpm there is an overriding parasympathetic drive acting on the heart without which the resting pulse would rise to around 90–100 bpm.

Factors affecting cardiac output include **heart rate, contractility, preload** and **afterload**. The contractility of the heart is a measure of cardiac performance for a given preload and afterload. The ejection fraction is the ratio of the volume of blood ejected from the left ventricle in each beat to the total amount of blood in the left ventricle at the end of diastole. It is the most widely used index of contractility.

Digoxin inhibits the Na/K/ATPase, increasing intracellular sodium which is exchanged for calcium resulting in an increased intracellular calcium concentration. This results in a positive inotropic effect.

11 Cardiac output:

A True
B True
C True
D True
E True

Cardiac output equals the product of heart rate and stroke volume. The heart rate is influenced by three important reflexes. The *baroreceptor reflex* responds to a drop in arterial pressure by increasing the heart rate. The *Bainbridge reflex* responds to an increase in venous return by increasing the heart rate. Various *respiratory reflexes* can also affect the heart rate either through the effect of hypocapnia (via chemoreceptors) or increased intrathoracic pressure (via mechanical stretch receptors) on the cardiac and respiratory centres in the pons and medulla.

The relationship between preload and stroke volume is explained by the Starling mechanism whereby an increase in preload results in an increase in stroke volume. Hence increasing the CVP results in an increase in cardiac output. However, an increase in cardiac output may result in a fall in CVP as explained by the vascular function curve. Therefore the precise relationship between cardiac output and venous pressure is a balance between the cardiac and vascular function curves.

Cardiac output is calculated by thermodilution or oesophageal Doppler.

12 The jugular venous pressure:
A False
B False
C True
D False
E True

The jugular venous pressure is the vertical height of the pulse in centimetres above the sternal angle and is an indicator of right atrial pressure. The waveform consists of an *a-wave* (atrial contraction), *c-wave* (tricuspid valve closure) and *v-wave* (end of ventricular systole). Causes of a **raised JVP** include exercise, expiration, right heart failure, fluid overload, bradycardia and cardiac tamponade (raised JVP on inspiration, Kussmaul's sign). **Cannon waves** are large a-waves with a rapid fall due to the atrium contracting against a closed tricuspid valve such as occurs in complete heart block, atrial flutter and ventricular tachycardia.

Absent a-waves are a feature of atrial fibrillation.

13 In the cardiac cycle:
A False
B False
C False
D False
E True

The *mitral valve* opens in diastole at the point of the *third heart sound*, and *closes* at the point of the first heart sound. The second heart sound occurs at the closure of the aortic and pulmonary valves. The c-wave of the JVP occurs in ventricular systole after the QRS complex. Left ventricular pressure approximates to aortic pressure whilst the aortic valve is open. After the peak of left ventricular and aortic pressures, the left ventricular pressure falls more rapidly than the fall in aortic pressure, thereby resulting in closure of the aortic valve. Left atrial pressure gradually increases after closure of the mitral valve to a peak just before it opens.

14 Atrial fibrillation may be associated with:
A True
B True
C False
D True
E True

Causes of atrial fibrillation include myocardial infarction and ischaemia, hypertension, mitral valve disease, hyperthyroidism, carcinoma of the bronchus, sarcoidosis, haemochromatosis, cardiomyopathy, atrial myxoma, constrictive pericarditis and pneumonia.

15 Regarding electrocardiographic abnormalities:
A False
B True
C False
D False
E True

Hypokalaemia — Small T waves, U wave
Hyperkalaemia — Tall T waves, wide QRS, absent P waves
Hypocalcaemia — Long Q–T interval
Hypercalcaemia — Short Q–T interval
ST elevation — Infarction, ventricular aneurysm, pericarditis
ST depression — Ischaemia, digoxin therapy
Digoxin — ST depression, inverted T wave (V5–V6, 'reverse tick' appearance)

Right axis deviation occurs in right ventricular hypertrophy or strain, cor pulmonale, pulmonary stenosis but not right bundle branch block. The cardiac axis is usually normal because there is normal depolarization of the larger left ventricle. **Left axis deviation** occurs in left ventricular hypertrophy or strain and left anterior hemiblock.

16 Complications of acute tubular necrosis include:

A True
B False
C True
D True
E True

The list of complications resulting from acute tubular necrosis is long and includes metabolic acidosis, hyperkalaemia, hypocalcaemia, infection, uraemia and disseminated intravascular coagulation eventually leading to multi-organ dysfunction syndrome (MODS). Pericarditis and impaired platelet function result from uraemia which also leads to confusion and muscle twitching. Pulmonary oedema and heart failure may also occur.

17 Dopamine:

A True
B True
C False
D True
E False

Dopamine has a renal effect at lower doses of up to 5 µg/kg/min via D1 and D2 receptors by causing local vasodilation and increased renal blood flow. At higher doses it resembles noradrenaline by acting as an α-agonist, but also with some β_1 effects resulting in an increased cardiac output. Dopamine also increases diuretic delivery to the distal tubule, has a direct effect on tubular function and *decreases* serum aldosterone concentration. There is a wide variation in response to dopamine between individuals in terms of the promotion of urine flow.

18 In the treatment of pulseless ventricular tachycardia:

A True
B False
C False
D True
E True

In ventricular fibrillation or pulseless ventricular tachycardia, early defibrillation using *un*synchronized shocks is essential (200 joules, 200 J, 360 J). This is followed by cardiopulmonary resuscitation, 1 mg of adrenaline given every 3 minutes and early intubation. Atropine is used in asystole or peri-arrest bradycardias. Synchronized shocks should only be used for cardioversion when there is a pulse.

19 Causes of hypertension include:

A True
B False
C True
D False
E True

Essential hypertension accounts for 95% of all cases. Causes of **secondary hypertension** include renal artery stenosis, glomerulonephritis, polycystic kidneys, polyarteritis nodosa, systemic sclerosis, Conn's syndrome, Cushing's syndrome, acromegaly, phaeochromocytoma, hyperparathyroidism and steroids.

20 In a lateral thoracotomy:

A False
B False
C True
D True
E False

Lateral thoracotomy may be *anterolateral* or *posterolateral* or a combination of both approaches. The anterolateral is through the fourth rib space, and is used for transaxillary sympathectomy. The posterolateral approach through the sixth rib space gives access to the lungs. Superficial muscles divided in the anterolateral approach include pectoralis major, pectoralis minor, serratus anterior and latissimus dorsi.

21 Regarding arterial lines:
A False
B True
C True
D True
E True

Arterial lines may be inserted into the femoral, radial, brachial and dorsalis pedis arteries. Hazards include haematoma formation, haemorrhage (especially on disconnection), true and false aneurysm formation, arterio-venous fistulae, distal ischaemia or infarction, local infection, septicaemia and anaemia. *Allen's test* is used to assess the collateral circulation in the hand by occlusion of the ulnar and radial arteries followed by release of each artery in turn.

22 Complications of tracheostomy include:
A True
B True
C True
D True
E True

There are a number of complications of **tracheostomy** which occur *during* the operation such as anoxia and haemorrhage, and those that occur in the *postoperative* period such as airway obstruction, surgical emphysema, infection and tracheo-oesophageal fistula. Tracheal stenosis is a *late* complication.

23 Causes of hilar enlargement include:
A True
B True
C False
D True
E False

Causes of **hilar lymphadenopathy** include pulmonary arterial hypertension and lymphadenopathy secondary to tuberculosis, sarcoid, lymphoma or metastases. Caplan's syndrome is the combination of rheumatoid arthritis and necrotic lung granulomata which results in bilateral lung but not hilar nodules on chest radiography.

24 Muscles involved in expiration during quiet breathing include:
A False
B False
C False
D False
E False

Expiration is passive during quiet breathing. During exertional expiration, muscles including rectus abdominis, internal intercostals and external oblique may be involved in forcefully expelling air from the thorax.

25 The following stimulate breathing via the respiratory centre:
A True
B False
C True
D True
E False

The respiratory centre in the pons and medulla exerts automatic control of breathing in terms of the depth and rate of inspiration as well as the timing of inspiration and expiration. A rise in the $PaCO_2$ causes a fall in the pH of the cerebrospinal fluid, thereby stimulating the central chemoreceptors which contribute towards the triggering of inspiratory activity. Baroreceptors, body temperature, proprioceptors and chemical agents have afferent inputs to the respiratory centre and therefore may affect the exact pattern of breathing. Yawning, swallowing, pain and sneezing may all influence respiration via higher CNS centres which include the cerebral cortex, limbic system and hypothalamus.

ANSWERS TO EXTENDED MATCHING QUESTIONS

Topic: Shock

1 D
2 C
3 A
4 B

Topic: Respiratory abnormalities

1 D

These figures are suggestive of an obstructive picture. The lungs are more compliant than normal and there is alveolar wall destruction. This usually leads to a reduced FEV_1:FVC ratio, increased RV and TLC and reduced transfer factor (DLCO).

2 B

This is suggestive of a restrictive pattern of lung disease. Inflammation thickens the alveolar membrane resulting in reduced compliance. Lung volumes and transfer factor are therefore low. The KCO can be maintained if the rest of the lung is normal.

Note: DLCO gas transfer factor reflects function at the alveolar capillary interface and depends on the lung volume sampled. KCO is the DLCO corrected for sampled lung volume and is therefore a more specific measure of alveolar capillary pathology. DLCO and KCO are both *decreased* in pneumonectomy, anaemia, childhood,

restrictive lung disease, COAD, pulmonary oedema and embolism, and are *increased* in exercise, polycythaemia and alveolar haemorrhage. Asthma may give rise to an *increased* DLCO and a normal KCO, whereas scleroderma or SLE may give rise to a *reduced* DLCO and a normal KCO (due to a loss of complete functional units).

Topic: Nutrition

1 F

There is no reason why this man needs anything more than routine perioperative hydration.

2 D

Needle catheter jejunostomy is the preferred method of enteral feeding in this case as feeding directly into the stomach may be hazardous in view of the surgical procedure being carried out.

3 A

Nasogastric feeding is a reasonable initial option in this young trauma victim although other forms of feeding may become more appropriate depending on her injuries and the treatment required for them. Nasojejunal feeding is an alternative.

4 E

This man ideally needs total bowel rest.

5: Neoplasia

1 Regarding cancer death rates over the last 50 years in the UK:

A Pancreatic cancer has increased

B Lung cancer in men has fallen

C Gastric cancer has increased

D Uterine cancer has fallen

E Colon cancer in women has fallen

2 Gastric cancer:

A Japan has amongst the poorest 5-year survival rates in the world

B Is associated with blood group O

C May present with a Krukenberg tumour

D Has a higher incidence in the lower social classes

E Is found in areas of gastritis in over 30% of cases

3 Cellular changes suggestive of malignant transformation include:

A Multiple nucleoli

B Mitotic figures

C An increase in the cytoplasmic : nuclear ratio

D Proliferation of stroma

E Hyperchromatism

4 Medullary carcinoma of the thyroid:

A Arises from parafollicular cells

B Typically secretes calcitonin

C Most cases are familial

D Is treated by total thyroidectomy with ipsilateral modified block dissection

E 5-year survival is over 50% in node negative cases

5 Colorectal carcinoma:

A Is the leading cause of cancer deaths in men and women

B Ureterosigmoidostomy is a risk factor

C Colon cancer is more common in women than in men

D 50% of cases occur in the sigmoid colon and rectum, and 50% in the caecum

E A synchronous carcinoma is found in about 5% of cases

6 A doctor may break confidentiality:

A In an NHS tribunal

B When instructed to by the Criminal Prosecution Service

C When respecting confidentiality places a named individual at risk of serious harm

D If the patient is a terrorist

E In reporting notifiable diseases

7 In the female breast:

A The glands are closely adherent to the pectoralis major muscle

B The blood supply is from the internal thoracic and axillary arteries

C Lymphatic drainage is continuous across the midline

D The bulk of the breast overlies the fourth to the eighth ribs

E Most lesions are benign

8 Risk factors for malignant melanoma include:

A Blue eyes

B Xeroderma pigmentosum

C Red hair

D Dysplastic naevus syndrome

E Continuous sun exposure

9 Regarding breast cancer:

A Histologically most cases are ductal carcinoma-in-situ

B Paget's disease occurs in 2% of cases

C Pain is a feature in up to 10% of cases

D   Mastectomy should be followed by
    radiotherapy
E   There is no difference in the 5-year
    survival or recurrence rate between
    mastectomy and wide local excision with
    radiotherapy

**10 Carcino-embryonic antigen is a useful
    marker for:**
A   Uterine adenocarcinoma
B   Prostate adenocarcinoma
C   Testicular seminomas
D   Medullary carcinoma of the thyroid
E   Germ cell ovarian tumours

**11 The following are macroscopic features
    of malignant neoplasms:**
A   Sessile lesion
B   Polyploid lesion
C   Ulcerated lesion
D   Papillary lesion
E   Fungating lesion

12 Lung cancer:
A   Of the alveolar cell type is not typically
    associated with smoking
B   Of the large cell type characteristically
    metastasizes early
C   May present with the myasthenic
    syndrome
D   Of the small cell type has the best 5-year
    survival of all types of lung cancer when
    treated by excision
E   May present with hypernatraemia due to
    hormone secretion by the tumour

13 Renal cancer may present with:
A   Pain
B   Pyrexia
C   A palpable mass as a late feature
D   Polycythaemia which occurs more
    commonly than anaemia
E   Hypocalcaemia

14 Regarding Hodgkin's disease:
A   Pel-Ebstein fever is a characteristic
    feature
B   Painful lymph nodes commonly occur
C   A staging laparotomy does not improve
    survival

D   Combination chemotherapy is given for
    all stages of B type lymphoma
E   The lymphocyte predominant subtype
    has a good prognosis

**15 Tumours which may be treated with
    radiotherapy include:**
A   Basal cell carcinomas
B   Brainstem gliomas
C   Malignant melanoma
D   Laryngeal carcinoma
E   Testicular seminoma

16 Tumour suppressor genes:
A   Increased gene product due to
    upregulation of the p53 tumour
    suppressor gene may be implicated in
    the development of breast cancer
B   Are implicated in the development of
    multiple colonic polyps and early
    colorectal cancer
C   Encode for nuclear and cytoplasmic
    proteins which are normally inhibitory
D   Loss of one allele of the Rb
    (retinoblastoma) gene is sufficient to give
    rise to retinoblastoma in familial cases
E   The C-myc tumour suppressor gene
    undergoes translocation from
    chromosome 8 to 14 in Burkitt's
    lymphoma

17 Regarding gastric cancer:
A   Antral lesions are more common than
    fundal lesions
B   It may present as a right supraclavicular
    node mass
C   Operative mortality at 30 days for a D2
    gastrectomy exceeds 25%
D   Gastric lymphoma is the commonest
    extranodal primary site for non-
    Hodgkin's lymphoma
E   Gastric leiomyosarcomas most often
    present with outlet obstruction

18 Tumour invasion:
A   Homotypic cell adhesion is due to
    desmosomes
B   Transforming growth factor β stimulates
    angiogenesis
C   Loss of E-cadherin promotes invasion

D Transforming growth factor α inhibits angiogenesis

E A negative charge on the surface of cells promotes adhesion

19 In the management of colorectal carcinoma:

A 50% of cases may be found on sigmoidoscopy

B Surgery should be avoided in patients with liver metastases

C The 5-year survival for a Dukes' B lesion is below 50%

D Dukes' C involves the presence of liver metastases

E Preoperative radiotherapy rarely affects resectability

20 Causes of pain in a breast include:

A A cyst

B Fibroadenosis

C An abscess

D Pregnancy mastitis

E A fibroadenoma

21 Causes of gynaecomastia include:

A Renal failure

B Oestrogen therapy

C Ranitidine

D Diuretics

E Carcinoma

22 Risk factors for breast cancer include:

A Late menarche

B Nulliparity

C Unopposed oestrogen therapy

D High saturated fat intake

E Benign atypical hyperplasia

23 Regarding malignant melanoma:

A The lentigo maligna variety has a good prognosis

B Breslow thickness is a better prognostic indicator than Clarke's levels

C Ulcerated lesions should be excised with a 3 cm margin

D Chemotherapy is useful for thick lesions

E Isolated limb perfusion is effective at reducing the size of a lesion

24 Screening for breast cancer:

A Occurs in women between 55 to 69 years of age

B Involves two-view mammography

C Has 85–95% accuracy for the detection of malignant lesions

D Has reduced mortality from breast cancer in the UK

E Results in increased early detection of tumours

25 The following tumours characteristically result in bone metastases:

A Breast carcinoma

B Renal adenocarcinoma

C Papillary carcinoma of the thyroid

D Colorectal carcinoma

E Prostate carcinoma

EXTENDED MATCHING QUESTIONS

Topic: Staging for breast carcinoma

A T1N1M0
B T1N2M0
C T2N3M0
D T2N2M0
E T2N1M0
F T3N2M1
G T4N1M0
H T4N2M0
I T4N2M1

For each case, select the most appropriate stage from the list of options above. Each option may be used once, more than once or not at all.

1 A 71-year-old woman with a 3 cm carcinoma in her right breast fixed to the chest wall with mobile nodes in the right axilla.
2 A 52-year-old woman with a 2.5 cm mobile carcinoma in her left breast with mobile nodes in the left axilla.
3 A 44-year-old woman with a 4 cm carcinoma in her right breast with skin fixity superiorly and fixed nodes in the right axilla.
4 A 57-year-old woman with an 8 cm mobile carcinoma in her left breast with fixed nodes in the left axilla and mobile nodes in the right axilla.

Topic: Bowel operations

A Left hemicolectomy
B Right hemicolectomy
C Abdomino-perineal resection
D Sigmoid colectomy
E Anterior resection
F Hartmann's procedure
G Defunctioning loop ileostomy
H Total colectomy
I No surgery

For each case, select the most appropriate operation from the list of options above. Each option may be used once, more than once or not at all.

1 A 46-year-old man presents to the accident and emergency department with lower abdominal pain, tachycardia, and leucocytosis. Peritonitis is diagnosed and at laparotomy, perforated diverticular disease of the sigmoid is seen.
2 A 57-year-old man presents to outpatients with a history of constipation. Rigid sigmoidoscopy reveals a constricting mass at 10 cm. Biopsies confirm adenocarcinoma. The location of the tumour is confirmed on the operating table.
3 A 68-year-old woman presents with intermittent constipation and diarrhoea, tenesmus and fresh rectal bleeding. A large mass is found very low in the rectum on digital examination. Ultrasound is suspicious of liver metastases.
4 A 62-year-old woman presents with iron deficiency anaemia and positive faecal occult blood. Barium enema reveals a lesion in the colon close to the ileocaecal junction.

Topic: Management of the terminally ill

A Radiotherapy
B Steroids
C Surgery
D Chemotherapy
E Non-steroidal anti-inflammatory agents
F Amitriptyline

For each scenario below, select the most appropriate treatment from the list of options above. Each option may be used once, more than once or not at all.

1 A tumour in the sigmoid colon causing obstruction with liver metastases.
2 A brain stem glioma.
3 A 70-year-old woman with an ulcerated and necrotic breast cancer causing widespread local destruction, together with malignant lymph nodes.

4 A patient with bilateral pubic rami fractures.

5 A patient with known ulcerative colitis presenting with profuse bloody diarrhoea. He is unwell, tachycardic with LIF tenderness and his transverse colon measures 8 cm in diameter on plain abdominal radiography.

ANSWERS TO MULTIPLE CHOICE QUESTIONS

1 Regarding cancer death rates over the last 50 years in the UK:

A True
B False
C False
D True
E True

In general, the overall **cancer mortality rate** has been increasing. Over the last fifty years mortality rates for lung cancer have increased at a very high rate in men and more recently in women. Pancreatic cancer has also increased. Stomach cancer has fallen heavily as have uterine and colon cancers in women. Most frequent sites for cancer death in men are lung, colorectal, prostate, pancreas and stomach. For women they are breast, lung, colorectal, ovary and uterus.

2 Gastric cancer:

A False
B False
C True
D True
E False

Gastric cancer is more common in Japan where detection occurs at an earlier stage than in the UK as a result of screening. Five-year survival in Japan is in excess of 50% compared with 5–10% in the UK. Chile and Finland also have increased death rates from gastric cancer. Risk factors include blood group A, lower social class, pernicious anaemia, a positive family history, polyps, atrophic gastritis, chronic biliary gastritis, partial gastrectomy and acanthosis nigricans. Over 90% of carcinomas are found in areas of gastritis.

3 Cellular changes suggestive of malignant transformation include:

A True
B False
C False
D True
E True

Malignant transformation is suggested by *growth changes* (lack of differentiation, uncontrolled proliferation, loss of contact inhibition) and *morphologic changes*. These include pleomorphism (variation in size and shape of cells), necrosis, cytoplasmic changes (increased cytoplasmic staining and abnormal cellular outlines) and nuclear changes. The latter tend to be the most predominant and include hyperchromatism (nucleus stains darkly), an increase in the nuclear : cytoplasmic ratio, chromatin clumping, large and often multiple nucleoli and the presence of large numbers of mitotic figures many of which have abnormal configurations. Mitotic figures are also seen in benign lesions but they tend to be fewer and normal in appearance. The stroma is the supportive connective tissue of a neoplasm and its proliferation is indicative of tumour invasion.

4 Medullary carcinoma of the thyroid:

A True
B True
C False
D True
E False

Medullary carcinoma of the thyroid accounts for 5–10% of thyroid neoplasms, with most being sporadic and some familial. It arises from the parafollicular cells and secretes many substances including calcitonin and carcino-embryonic antigen. Some patients may present with diarrhoea. About one-quarter of patients have lymph node metastases at presentation. Calcitonin is a useful marker for the detection of recurrence after total thyroidectomy. Ipsilateral modified block dissection is performed for patients whatever the node status, although bilateral block dissection is carried out for patients with multicentric disease. Five-year survival is quoted as being 90% in node-negative patients and 50% in node-positive patients.

5 Colorectal carcinoma:
A False
B True
C True
D False
E True

Colorectal cancer is the second highest cause of cancer deaths in men and the third highest in women, resulting in about 20 000 deaths every year. Colon cancer is more common in women and rectal cancer is more common in men. Roughly one-half of the tumours are in the rectum, one-quarter in the sigmoid colon and the remainder mainly in the caecum with 5–10% in the rest of the colon. A second cancer is found in about 5% of cases. Macroscopically the cancer is usually polypoidal or ulcerating, the former more common in right sided lesions and the latter in rectal lesions. Although not often performed for urinary diversion, ureterosigmoidostomy is a risk factor for the development of colorectal carcinoma presumably due to the carcinogenic properties of various urinary constituents. Previous cholecystectomy has often been cited as a risk factor particularly for right sided lesions but there is no conclusive evidence.

6 A doctor may break confidentiality:
A True
B False
C True
D True
E True

A doctor *must* break confidentiality under certain circumstances including a court order or by a court judge, in reporting notifiable diseases, when giving evidence to an NHS tribunal and when a patient is suspected of terrorism within the UK. Breaking confidentiality is *discretionary* in circumstances where there may be evidence of a criminal risk to others, a threat to others, or the risk of serious harm or death to a named individual.

7 In the female breast:
A False
B True
C True
D False
E True

The female breast overlies the second to the sixth ribs, lying on pectoralis major and serratus anterior. The retromammary space separates the breast from pectoralis major. Blood supply is from the axillary artery via its lateral thoracic and acromiothoracic branches, perforating branches of the internal thoracic artery and lateral perforating branches of the intercostal arteries. Venous drainage is to the corresponding veins. Lymphatic drainage of the lateral part of the breast is to the axilla, and of the medial breast to the internal mammary chain although there are connections between the two lymph node groups. Lymph may also drain from one breast to the other due to connections across the midline. Axillary lymph nodes include anterior, posterior, lateral, central and apical groups.

8 Risk factors for malignant melanoma include:
A True
B True
C True
D True
E False

Risk factors for malignant melanoma also include fair skin, blond hair syndrome, albinism and previous melanoma. Melanomas are typically associated with *intermittent* sun exposure, whereas basal and squamous cell carcinomas are associated with *continuous* sun exposure.

9 Regarding breast cancer:
A False
B True
C True
D False
E False

About 80–90% of breast carcinomas are of the invasive ductal epithelial type and 2% of the invasive lobular type. Up to 5% are ductal carcinoma-in-situ and 1% lobular carcinoma-in-situ. Two per cent are associated with Paget's disease in which an intraductal carcinoma spreads within the epithelium to the skin of the nipple and into the substance of the breast. The least aggressive tumours are non-invasive intraductal and lobular carcinoma in-situ (LCIS) both of which rarely metastasize. Skin changes may be very similar to eczema including reddening, weeping, formation of crust but rarely itching. Hence, women with such presentations must be investigated despite the absence of any palpable lump. Up to 20% of cases present as advanced disease.

For mobile carcinomas, trials indicate no difference in the 5-year survival rate between mastectomy or breast conservation and radiotherapy. Local recurrence is, however, increased if breast conservation is employed which includes wide local excision, lumpectomy or quadrantectomy. Radiotherapy after a mastectomy with axillary clearance gives rise to an increased incidence of arm lymphoedema which otherwise affects 5% of women.

The presence of oestrogen receptor positivity (ER$^+$) reflects better tumour differentiation and thus a potentially better response to hormonal manipulation. Tumours which are ER$^+$ are likely to be progesterone receptor positive (PR$^+$) as well. If a tumour is PR$^+$ but ER negative (ER$^-$) it has a worse prognosis than if PR$^-$/ER$^+$.

10 Carcino-embryonic antigen is a useful marker for:

A True
B True
C False
D True
E False

Carcino-embryonic antigen (CEA) is a marker for many tumours including uterine adenocarcinoma, prostate adenocarcinoma, medullary carcinoma of the thyroid, breast adenocarcinoma, adenocarcinoma and small-cell carcinoma of the lung, colorectal adenocarcinoma, pancreas and stomach adenocarcinoma. β **Human chorionic gonadotrophin** is a marker for testicular seminoma, uterine choriocarcinoma and ovarian germ cell tumours.

11 The following are macroscopic features of malignant neoplasms:

A True
B False
C True
D False
E True

Neoplasms which are sessile, fungating, ulcerating and annular constricting lesions in a hollow muscular organ are more likely to be malignant. Polyploid and papillary lesions are generally benign features.

12 Lung cancer:

A False
B True
C True
D False
E False

Lung cancer is the leading cause of cancer deaths in the UK. The major risk factor is smoking, but others include asbestos, radioactivity, chromium and iron.
Adenocarcinomas are peripheral tumours which are characteristically not related to smoking but can be associated with asbestos exposure. Squamous cell carcinoma is the most common type and is radiosensitive. Small cell carcinomas are usually disseminated at presentation, and may present with paraneoplastic syndromes. Inappropriate secretion of antidiuretic hormone causes *hypo*natraemia. Large cell carcinomas are less well differentiated and metastasize early. Alveolar cell carcinomas are rare, and are associated with chronic inflammation and smoking.

13 Renal cancer may present with:
A True
B True
C True
D False
E False

Renal cell carcinoma (hypernephroma) is more common in men and presents with loin pain, haematuria and a palpable mass although this classic triad occurs in less than 10% of cases. Mass effect is a late feature, and other symptoms of weight loss and fever may occur. Associated features include hypertension due to renin secretion, hypercalcaemia due to parathyroid-like hormone secretion, hyponatraemia or nephrotic syndrome and erythrocytosis due to erythropoietin-like hormone. Anaemia may occur due to chronic loss of blood in the urine which on balance is more common than erythrocytosis.

14 Regarding Hodgkin's disease:
A True
B False
C True
D True
E True

Hodgkin's lymphoma presents with enlarged *painless* lymph nodes, usually in the neck or axillae. One-quarter have 'B' symptoms of fever, weight loss, night sweats, pruritis and malaise. *Pel-Ebstein fever* may occur where fever alternates with long periods of normal or low temperature. Staging laparotomy and splenectomy are being replaced by CT scanning. There is also the risk of post-splenectomy sepsis. Combined chemotherapy is recommended for all patients with 'B' symptoms. Out of the four types, lymphocyte depleted has the lowest incidence but the poorest prognosis, with lymphocyte predominant having the best prognisis.

15 Tumours which may be treated with radiotherapy include:
A True
B True
C False
D True
E True

Radiotherapy is used for radiosensitive tumours such as testicular seminomas, basal cell and squamous cell carcinomas, inoperable or difficult access areas such as brainstem gliomas, for functional preservation such as in the treatment of laryngeal cancer (voice is sacrificed with surgery), and in patients not fit for theatre.

16 Tumour suppressor genes:
A False
B True
C True
D False
E False

Tumour suppressor genes encode for nuclear, cytoplasmic and membrane bound proteins which normally contribute to the inhibition of cell proliferation. Mutations in or loss of these genes result in loss of inhibition of cell proliferation thereby promoting oncogenesis. **Oncogenes** are also found in the normal human genome when they are known as *proto-oncogenes*. They may become abnormally activated in one of several ways: either the gene is upregulated resulting in increased amounts of the normal gene product, or point mutations result in the formation of large amounts of an abnormal gene product, or fusion between parts of two proto-oncogenes occurs usually secondary to chromosomal translocation and resulting in a new gene product. The tumour suppressor gene p53 is implicated in breast and other cancers in which there is either complete loss of expression of the p53 gene or a mutation resulting in a new gene product, but *not* overexpression of p53 as this is a characteristic of dominantly acting oncogenes. The **familial adenomatous polyposis coli (FAP)** and **deleted in colon**

cancer (DCC) genes are both tumour suppressor genes implicated in the development of familial polyposis and colorectal cancer. In retinoblastoma, the loss of or mutations in *two* alleles of the **Rb gene** are required before retinoblastoma results. In familial cases, one of these mutations may be inherited thus only one spontaneous somatic mutation is required in life to result in disease. **Burkitt's lymphoma** results from a translocation of the c-myc *proto-oncogene* from chromosome 8 to chromosome 14.

17 Regarding gastric cancer:

A True
B False
C False
D True
E False

Antral lesions are more common than fundal lesions and tend to cause gastric outflow obstruction, whereas lesions in the *cardia* cause dysphagia and *fundal* lesions present late with anaemia. Troisier's sign is a *left* supraclavicular node mass (Virchow's node) suggesting advanced disease.

A **D2 gastrectomy** (previously known as R2) involves removal of N1 and N2 nodes with a 5 cm clearance of the tumour and carries an operative mortality of 5% or less. This is the operation of choice in Japan where detailed nodal assessment and sampling has improved survival.

Gastric lymphoma is the commonest extranodal primary site for non-Hodgkin's lymphoma, and is treated with resection, chemotherapy and radiotherapy. Gastric leiomyosarcomas most often present with haemorrhage and occur either *de novo* or from a leiomyoma.

18 Tumour invasion:

A True
B False
C True
D False
E True

The formation of **metastases** involves a series of events in which tumour cellular deposits travel to sites distant from their origin (in many ways similar to vascular embolism) where they establish their own blood supply and rapidly flourish. This process involves a decrease in homotypic tumour cell adhesion which is normally promoted by the presence of desmosomes, negative cell surface charge and cadherins. Hence the loss of E-cadherin or E-cadherin antibodies promote invasion. *Tumour autocrine motility factor (AMF)* and *scatter factor* are also thought to promote shedding of cells from the primary tumour mass. Subsequent invasion into blood vessels or lymphatics is aided by *cadherins* and *proteases* in particular type IV gelatinase. *Tissue inhibitors of protease activity (TIMPs)* have been found to be expressed on the long arm of chromosome 17. This is the same site as the *NM23 gene,* the expression of which is associated with a good prognosis in human breast cancer. Following transfer to a distant site, cell adhesion molecules including integrins bind to basement membrane components such as laminin and fibronectin. Angiogenesis followed by multiplication then occurs. Signals promoting angiogenesis include basic fibroblast growth factor, angiogenin and transforming growth factor α. Transforming growth factor β and angiostatin inhibit angiogenesis.

19 In the management of colorectal carcinoma:

A True
B False
C False
D False
E False

With the majority of **colorectal carcinomas** being in the rectum and sigmoid colon, over 50% may be found on sigmoidoscopy. Surgery is palliative when liver metastases are present, and may play a part in reducing obstruction and symptoms such as rectal bleeding. **Preoperative radiotherapy** is being used at centres for downgrading lower rectal tumours, thereby improving resectability. Dukes' A tumours are confined to the bowel wall, Dukes' B penetrate through the wall, Dukes' C involve local nodes and Dukes' D has been added for distant metastases. Survival rates have improved with 5-year survival at 80–90% for Dukes' A, 60–70% for Dukes' B, 30–50% for Dukes' C and below 10% for Dukes' D.

20 Causes of pain in a breast include:
A True
B True
C True
D True
E False

Painful breast lumps include fibroadenosis, cysts, abscesses, periductal mastitis and rarely carcinoma. Fibroadenomas are typically *painless* rubbery smooth lumps occurring in younger women, nicknamed 'breast mouse' due to their mobility. Mastalgia and pregnancy mastitis are other causes of painful breasts. Carcinomas tend to be painless, irregular and hard lumps. Pregnancy is the commonest cause of changes in the breast.

21 Causes of gynaecomastia include:
A True
B True
C False
D True
E False

Male breast enlargement or **gynaecomastia** has an increase in the ductal and connective tissue elements of the breast, but not in the number of lobules. It may occur in neonates and in puberty and old age. The texture may be soft or hard and enlargement may occur in one or both breasts. Gynaecomastia may follow hormone secreting neoplasms, hypogonadism, liver and renal disease. Many drugs may also cause gynaecomastia and include spironolactone, cimetidine, digoxin, metoclopramide, diuretics and oestrogens.

22 Risk factors for breast cancer include:
A False
B True
C True
D True
E True

Breast cancer is the commonest cause of cancer deaths in women and affects about 1 in 12 women. It increases with increasing age. Risk factors include nulliparity, early menarche and late menopause, oestrogen therapy unopposed by progesterone, positive family history, saturated fat intake and previous benign atypical hyperplasia. Breastfeeding and an early first child are both protective.

23 Regarding malignant melanoma:
A True
B True
C True
D False
E True

Types of **malignant melanoma** include *superficial spreading* which is the most common type (60–70%), *nodular, acral lentiginous* and *lentigo maligna*. Lentigo has the best prognosis and is the least aggressive with slow growth. Nodular and acral lentiginous have the worst prognosis. **Breslow thickness** is the best prognostic factor although **Clark's level** may also be used. A combination of tumour thickness, level of invasion and nodal status is sometimes used. Other prognostic factors include *site of tumour* (scalp, hands and feet have a poorer prognosis), *age* (older patients have a worse prognosis), *gender* (women have a better prognosis than men although this in part may be due to the location of the tumour, in that women tend to get truncal lesions and men distal lesions) and *histological features* such as high mitotic rate. Ulcerated lesions require the biggest margin with 3 cm recommended. Malignant melanoma is sensitive to radiotherapy but not to chemotherapy. Agents are used in combination with isolated limb perfusion mainly for recurrences as this technique shrinks and may even completely heal lesions.

24 Screening for breast cancer:
A False
B True
C True
D False
E True

The UK National Breast Screening Programme originally offered single-view mammography but now includes two-view mammography for all women screened for the first time. It is offered to women between 50 and 64 years of age. The two views are superoinferior (SI) and mediolateral oblique (MLO). No definite increase in survival has been shown in the UK with this screening program which has shown benefit in Holland and Sweden. Mammography is the most sensitive and specific method of breast cancer screening and has increased early detection of tumours many of which are not palpable clinically.

25 The following tumours characteristically result in bone metastases:
A True
B True
C False
D False
E True

Prostate, lung, breast and kidney tumours commonly metastasize to bone. Papillary carcinoma of the thyroid spreads to local and regional lymph nodes, whereas follicular thyroid cancer spreads predominantly via the blood stream and may metastasize to bone. Lung, breast, kidney and thyroid lesions tend to be osteolytic whereas prostate secondaries are usually osteosclerotic. Colorectal carcinoma spreads mainly to the liver and lung.

Topic: Staging for breast carcinoma

1 G
2 E
3 H
4 F

The TNM classification of breast cancer is given below:

Tis	Carcinoma-in-situ/Paget's
T1	≥ 2 cm
T2	> 2 cm – < 5 cm
T3	> 5 cm
T4a	Chest wall extension (fixed)
T4b	Skin involvement
T4c	Both 4a and 4b
N0	No nodal involvement
N1	Ipsilateral axillary (mobile)
N2	Ipsilateral axillary (fixed)
N3	Ipsilateral internal mammary nodes
M0	No metastases
M1	Distant metastases

Topic: Bowel operations

1 F

In the presence of faecal peritonitis, bowel anastomosis is strongly discouraged owing to the risk of subsequent anastomotic dehiscence. A Hartmann's procedure is therefore recommended in the initial phase, and reversal of the end colostomy can take place at a later stage.

2 E

An anterior resection is the elective procedure of choice with a high tumour that has enough distal rectum to make a direct anastomosis feasible. If the tumour is situated more proximally such as in the sigmoid colon, a sigmoid colectomy may be performed.

3 C

An A-P resection is indicated, even in the presence of liver metastases as the patient may otherwise obstruct.

4 B

A right hemicolectomy would be the elective procedure of choice.

Topic: Management of the terminally ill

1 C

Surgery is indicated to relieve acute bowel obstruction secondary to a tumour even in the presence of liver metastases.

2 A

Surgery to remove the glioma is hazardous in this region of the brain, thus radiotherapy is the preferred option.

3 C

In this case surgery is required to control advanced local disease but will not improve the overall prognosis.

4 E

This type of fracture rarely requires surgical intervention unless associated with more extensive pelvic injuries. Effective analgesia is an important part of rapid recovery.

5 C

Most patients with exacerbations of their colitis can be adequately managed with aggressive medical therapy including local and systemic steroids. This patient presents with features suggestive of toxic megacolon (tachycardia, tenderness on abdominal examination and a colon in excess of 6 cm on abdominal radiograph) which are indications for prompt surgical intervention.

Section 2
Systems Modules

A: Locomotor

MULTIPLE CHOICE QUESTIONS

1 The humerus:
A Supracondylar fractures may be complicated by cubitus valgus
B Forms the medial boundary of the quadrilateral space
C Gives origin to infraspinatus from the lesser tuberosity
D Flexion may occur by the action of muscles innervated by the axillary nerve
E Shoulder dislocation may cause loss of sensation over the upper half of deltoid

2 Colles' fractures:
A Are associated with an intra-articular element
B Are associated with carpal tunnel syndrome
C May be associated with rupture of flexor pollicis longus
D Always involve the radius and ulna
E Are less common in patients on hormone replacement therapy

3 The cephalic vein:
A Begins in the anatomical snuff box
B Is at risk in the delto-pectoral approach to the humerus
C Has no valves
D Passes through the clavipectoral fascia with the lateral thoracic artery
E Can be used in emergency venous cut-down

4 Dermatomes:
A C1 has no representation on the skin
B T1 is not represented in the palm
C T2 supplies the axilla
D C5 and T2 are reflected on the chest
E C7 supplies the middle finger

5 Paget's disease:
A Below the age of 85 is more common in men than women
B Is seen most often in Africans
C Deafness is a feature
D Patients usually have high plasma calcium levels
E Treatment of osteosarcoma is more successful in these patients

6 Fractures of the neck of femur:
A Patients with osteoarthritis are more likely to get extracapsular fractures
B If intracapsular and partly displaced is classified as Garden II
C If Garden IV presenting within 6 hours of injury may be treated by AO screw fixation
D The risk of avascular necrosis in Garden IV fractures is less than 40%
E The proximal fragment may be flexed by iliacus and abducted by gluteus medius and minimus

7 The medial meniscus of the knee:
A Gives attachment posteriorly to the tendon of popliteus
B Peripheral tears usually do not heal
C Tears are associated with swelling which usually appears immediately
D Pain is more ill-defined compared with lateral meniscal tears
E Locking suggests a bucket-handle rather than anterior horn tear

8 The Trendelenberg sign:
A Is positive in congenital dislocation of the hip
B Is said to be positive if the pelvis drops on the side ipsilateral to the weak abductors

C If positive may be caused by fractured neck of femur

D Standing on the right leg may cause the left hip to droop if there is damage to the right inferior gluteal nerve

E May be positive in a painful hip due to a loose body

9 Compartment syndrome:

A Is more common in proximal than distal tibial fractures

B A pulse may be present

C Intracompartmental pressure measurements are commonly used in diagnosis

D Active hyperextension of the fingers is a useful clinical sign

E Treatment involves removal of tight plaster casts and prompt reduction of fractures

10 At the ankle:

A Talar shift indicates damage to the inferior tibio-fibular joint.

B Flexor hallucis longus is medial to flexor digitorum longus

C The short saphenous vein lies anterior to the lateral malleolus

D The skin over the medial malleolus is supplied by a branch of the femoral nerve

E The fibula transmits 40% of body weight through the ankle in normal subjects

11 The following are features of rheumatoid arthritis:

A Approximately 50% will have polyarticular involvement at onset

B Ulnar deviation at the metacarpophalangeal joints does not usually develop until more than one year from time of onset of the disease

C Vertebral artery occlusion

D Hoarseness of voice

E Pleural effusion

12 Osteoarthritis:

A If secondary, is usually polyarticular

B If primary generalized, has an equal sex distribution

C An early radiological feature includes subchondral cyst formation

D Perthe's disease is a predisposing condition

E The incidence is reduced in people taking analgesics

13 In total hip replacement:

A The posterior approach is associated with a lower rate of dislocations than the anterior approach

B The posterior approach involves division of gluteus medius and minimus to expose the capsule

C Bleeding during the anterior approach usually originates from the lateral circumflex femoral artery

D Anteversion of the acetabular cup is less desirable than retroversion

E Patients should not bear weight for 3–4 days postoperatively owing to the risk of dislocation

14 In the foot:

A Eversion is increased in plantar flexion

B Eversion is limited by tension in the deltoid ligament

C The medial longitudinal arch has flexor hallucis longus as its main support

D The lateral longitudinal arch has peroneus brevis as its main support

E The sural nerve supplies the skin over the heel

15 Amputations:

A Early weight bearing at 2–3 days postoperatively should be encouraged after below knee amputations

B Osteoarthritis of the knee is a contraindication to below knee amputations

C Inspection of flap bleeding at the time of operation is not as good as preoperative oximetry in determining the likely success of a below knee amputation

D Arteriovenous fistula is a recognized complication

E Muscle herniation may occur

16 Congenital dislocation of the hip:

A Can be distinguished from traumatic dislocation by the slope of the acetabulum on an X-ray

B Has an equal sex distribution

C Tends to be more common on the left side

D Oligohydramnios is a predisposing factor

E Ultrasound is usually used to demonstrate an effusion in high risk infants

17 Cervical vertebrae:

A The vertebral artery ascends behind the anterior rami of the cervical nerves

B Vertebrae 3 to 7 are typical

C 25% of the weight of the skull is transmitted through the dens to the axis

D Neck pain from a prolapsed intervertebral disc may be due to pressure on the posterior longitudinal ligament

E Paraesthesia from a prolapsed intervertebral disc is rarely bilateral

18 The shoulder:

A Its nerve supply includes the musculocutaneous nerve

B Part of the nerve supply to teres major and deltoid originates from the same nerve

C The long head of triceps is attached to the infraglenoid tubercle

D The rotator cuff muscles are all supplied by the posterior cord of the brachial plexus

E The profunda brachii artery passes through the quadrilateral space with the axillary nerve

19 Disorders of the shoulder:

A Pain with complete rotator cuff tears characteristically subsides more rapidly than with partial tears

B Painful arc with the impingement syndrome is less severe when the shoulder is abducted in a position of lateral rotation

C All complete tears should be surgically repaired

D Adhesive capsulitis may mimic reflex sympathetic dystrophy

E In adhesive capsulitis stiffness usually precedes the pain

20 In the region of the elbow:

A The brachial artery bifurcates at the level of the elbow joint

B Forced extension of the wrist may help in reaching a diagnosis of golfer's elbow

C A fractured medial epicondyle may cause weakness of pinch grip between the index finger and thumb

D Capsule of the elbow joint is attached to the head of the radius

E During arthroscopy insertion of the anteromedial port may damage the posterior interosseous nerve

21 Metabolic bone disease:

A Osteomalacia may present with carpopedal spasm

B The radiological changes of hyperparathyroidism may be seen in osteomalacia

C Alkaline phosphatase is normal in both osteoporosis and osteomalacia

D Thyrotoxicosis may predispose to osteoporosis

E Treatment of osteoporosis with bisphosphonates should be discontinued if fractures occur

22 Radial nerve:

A Division at the midshaft of the humerus causes weakness of elbow extension

B Pierces the lateral intermuscular septum to reach the anterior compartment of the arm

C Gives off two separate branches to the medial head of triceps

D Wrist drop without sensory impairment may be due to a lesion of the posterior interosseous nerve

E Palsy due to a fractured humerus needs to be surgically explored

23 Dupuytren's disease:

A Presenting in 60 to 70-year-olds is associated with a lower likelihood of

recurrence than in 30 to 40-year-olds
B The index and middle fingers are most commonly affected
C Is associated with fibromatosis of the plantar fascia
D Joint arthrodesis is a recognized treatment option
E Is associated with increased xanthine oxidase activity

24 Compression of the:
A Ulnar nerve may occur at the wrist
B Ulnar nerve eventually produces weakness of all the intrinsic muscles of the hand
C Ulnar nerve may produce weakness of flexion of the distal interphalangeal joint

D Median nerve at the wrist is most reliably elicited by testing flexor rather than abductor pollicis brevis
E Deep peroneal nerve due to a fracture of the fibula would cause an inability to evert the foot

25 Carpal tunnel syndrome:
A Is associated with haemophilia
B May cause pain in the shoulder
C The thumb and index finger are often spared from pain
D Weakness of thumb opposition is rarely a complication of surgical decompression
E Postoperatively the wrist is usually splinted in a position of slight extension

EXTENDED MATCHING QUESTIONS

Topic: Paraesthesia

A Prolapsed intervertebral disc at C6
B Cervical spondylosis
C Carpal tunnel syndrome
D Thoracic outlet syndrome
E Cervical tumour
F Rheumatoid arthritis

For each case scenario, select the most likely diagnosis from the list of options above. Each option may be used once, more than once or not at all.

1 A 40-year-old lady with a 3 year history of pain in both hands presents with upper motor neurone signs in her legs.
2 A 51-year-old man presents with a 2 month history of clumsiness. Examination reveals tenderness over the posterior neck muscles, with numbness and weakness localized to the C7 nerve root.
3 A 37-year-old female presents with intermittent pain in both forearms worse at night.
4 A 40-year-old male presents with pain on the ulnar border of his right hand and a lump on the ipsilateral side of his neck.

Topic: Knee pain

A Medial meniscal tear
B Posterior cruciate ligament rupture
C Anterior cruciate ligament rupture
D Osteoarthritis
E Sepsis
F Medial collateral ligament rupture

For each case scenario, select the most likely diagnosis from the list of options above. Each option may be used once, more than once or not at all.

1 A 20-year-old male presents with tenderness along the medial joint line following a rotational injury to his lower leg.

2 A 37-year-old male has pain on walking especially going downstairs.
3 A 40-year-old male presents with an effusion following a sports related injury to the knee. Examination reveals tenderness along the medial joint line. No ligamentous laxity is demonstrable on knee extension, but some mediolateral movement can be elicited when the knee is flexed by 30 degrees.

Topic: Bony lesions

A Metastasis
B Giant cell tumour
C Osteochondroma
D Ewing's tumour
E Osteoarthritis
F Osteosarcoma
G Osteoporosis

For each case scenario, select the most likely diagnosis from the list of options above. Each option may be used once, more than once or not at all.

1 A 60-year-old man with Paget's disease develops constant pain in his right knee.
2 A 21-year-old female presents with a mass in the mid shaft of her right femur 5 months after she was found to have an adrenal neuroblastoma.
3 An 18-year-old woman is found to have a suspicious looking lesion at the edge of the epiphyseal plate in the proximal end of her left humerus. The overlying cortex is not thinned.
4 A 52-year-old woman presents with pain in her back after falling down three steps. She underwent a hysterectomy and bilateral salpingo-oophorectomy at age 39.

ANSWERS TO MULTIPLE CHOICE QUESTIONS

1 The humerus:

A False
B False
C False
D True
E True

Supracondylar fractures commonly occur in children and are usually the result of a fall onto the outstretched hand. The structures passing through the cubital fossa are at risk of compression by displacement of the distal fragment posteriorly, although anterior displacement is also described. Clinical examination should therefore include assessment of median nerve function and presence of pulses. Malunion is a complication which may result in a *cubitus varus* deformity, which if marked requires supracondylar osteotomy.

The humerus forms the *lateral* boundary of the quadrilateral space and one of the triangular spaces as shown in Table 2.

The origin and insertion of the **rotator cuff muscles** is shown in Table 3.

The **axillary nerve** arises from the posterior cord of the brachial plexus (C5 and 6) and divides into anterior and posterior

Table 2

		Triangular 1	Triangular 2	Quadrilateral
Boundaries	Superior	Teres minor	Teres major	Teres minor
	Inferior	Teres major	—	Teres major
	Medial	—	Long head triceps	Long head triceps
	Lateral	Long head triceps	Humerus	Humerus
Contents	Nerve	—	Radial	Axillary
	Artery	Circumflex scapular	Profunda brachii	Posterior circumflex humeral

Table 3

	Origin	Insertion	Nerve supply
Infraspinatus	Infraspinous fossa of scapula	Greater tuberosity of humerus	Suprascapular nerve
Supraspinatus	Supraspinous fossa of scapula	Greater tuberosity	Suprascapular nerve
Teres minor	Upper two-thirds lateral border scapula	Greater tuberosity	Axillary nerve
Subscapularis	Subscapular fossa	Lesser tuberosity	Upper and lower subscapular nerves

divisions deep to deltoid. It supplies deltoid, teres minor, the skin over the lower half of deltoid and the upper lateral cutaneous nerve of arm.

2 Colles' fractures:
A False
B True
C False
D False
E True

Abraham Colles originally described in 1814 a transverse fracture of the distal radius with dorsal displacement of the distal fragment occurring in elderly people. Intra-articular extension and fracture of the ulna styloid process are other associated features but do not occur in all Colles' fractures. Typically elderly women with osteoporotic bone are affected, usually following a fall on the outstretched hand. The radial fragment is:
• dorsally displaced
• dorsally angulated
• radially displaced
• radially angulated.
There may be impaction or comminution.

Treatment involves
• *Reduction* This may not be necessary if the fracture is undisplaced but otherwise requires manipulation under anaesthesia
• *Immobilization* Usually with a plaster cast or well fitting dorsal slab
• *Rehabilitation* X-ray at 7–10 days to check for redisplacement; cast for 6 weeks

Complications
• Carpal tunnel syndrome
• Rupture of extensor pollicis longus. This tendon hooks around the dorsal tubercle of the radius (Lister's tubercle), and is supplied by branches of the anterior interosseous artery. Their occlusion after Colles' fractures may lead to necrosis and subsequent rupture of the tendon, causing a hammer thumb. This usually occurs a few weeks after the fracture, and may require tendon transfer from extensor indicis

• Malunion
• Stiffness
• Reflex sympathetic dystrophy or algodystrophy

3 The cephalic vein:
A True
B True
C False
D False
E True

The cephalic vein begins in the anatomical snuff box as a continuation of the radial side of the dorsal venous network. It ascends along the preaxial (radial) border of the forearm, becomes lateral to biceps in the deltopectoral groove and perforates the clavipectoral fascia to enter the axillary vein.

Structures passing through the **clavipectoral fascia**:

From superficial to deep
• Cephalic vein
• Lymphatic vessels

From deep to superficial
• Lateral pectoral nerve
• Thoraco-acromial artery

Uses for this vein: cutdown, Cimino fistula

4 Dermatomes:
A True
B True
C True
D False
E True

T1 has a motor supply in the hand but no sensory supply. The sensory component of T1 supplies the skin of the armpit and medial side of the arm through the medial cutaneous nerve of the arm.

The **sensory supply of C5** is represented over the lower half of the deltoid muscle by the upper lateral cutaneous nerve of the arm (upper half by the supraclavicular nerves and branches of the axillary nerve). It is not represented on the chest.

The **intercostobrachial nerve** is the lateral cutaneous branch of the second intercostal nerve. It extends to supply skin on the medial side of the upper arm, alongside the contribution by T1 and is occasionally supplemented by the lateral cutaneous branch of the third intercostal nerve.

5 Paget's disease:

A False
B False
C True
D False
E False

Paget's disease affects men and women equally. Most patients are asymptomatic. Over the age of 85 it is slightly more common in men than women. It is rare in Africans and relatively common in Britain, Germany and Australia. It is characterized by enlargement and thickening of the bone, but the internal architecture is normal.

Complications include fractures in weight bearing long bones, nerve compression and spinal stenosis, high output cardiac failure and osteosarcoma. Biochemical abnormalities usually include raised alkaline phosphatase (ALP) with normal plasma calcium and phosphate. Hypercalcaemia is a feature if the patient is immobilized. Treatment of osteosarcoma is less successful in patients with Paget's disease than in isolated cases.

6 Fractures of the neck of femur:

A True
B False
C True
D True
E False

In general, patients with osteoarthritis are more likely to suffer extracapsular fractures than intracapsular. This is because when the patient falls onto his hip, the reduced range of movement between the ball and socket prevents undue rotation of the proximal femur within the acetabulum. The force of landing on the greater tuberosity causes a fracture at the point of maximum impact, below the level of the femoral neck. As the femoral head is not at risk of avascular necrosis, such patients tend to be treated by dynamic hip screw fixation. Such patients in general tend to be older than those suffering intracapsular fractures.

Intracapsular fractures can be further subdivided according to the Garden classification:

I   Fracture through part of the femoral neck
II   Fracture through the whole of the femoral neck with no displacement
III Fracture with partial displacement of the femoral head
IV   Fracture with complete displacement of the femoral head

The higher the grade, the higher the risk of avascular necrosis of the femoral head. Hence it is commonly stated that patients with Garden III or IV fractures should undergo hemiarthroplasty, whereas those with Garden I or II fractures should undergo screw fixation to preserve the femoral head. However if a Garden IV fracture is fixed by AO screws within 12 hours of injury, the risk of avascular necrosis is around 20%, rising to 40% if perfomed after 24 hours (and almost 100% if left untreated). Thus it is reasonable to consider screw fixation in situations where the patient is likely to benefit from retaining their own femoral head, such as patients below the age of 65 or those previously active and mobile.

Flexion of the proximal fragment by iliacus and abduction by gluteus medius and minimus will only occur if the fracture occurs distal to the level of insertion of these muscles. Iliacus inserts just below the lesser trochanter of the femur, and gluteus medius and minimus insert into the greater trochanter. Thus fractures of the neck of femur are unlikely to produce movement of the proximal fragment, but a fracture of the *shaft* of the femur may cause such movement as described.

7 The medial meniscus of the knee:
A False
B False
C False
D False
E True

The tendon of **popliteus** inserts into the lateral surface of the lateral condyle of the femur, and also into the posterior part of the lateral meniscus. From the fully extended position, popliteus causes lateral rotation of the femur on the tibia to enable unlocking of the knee joint, but further lateral rotation of the femur is only possible once the lateral meniscus has been drawn posteriorly over the posterior margin of the lateral tibial condyle, again by the action of popliteus.

    Menisci in general are avascular but peripherally may receive a blood supply from the surrounding capsule, thus peripheral tears heal more readily than central ones. The swelling following a meniscal tear is not usually present at the time of the injury, characteristically appearing over the course of several hours. Medial meniscal tears cause pain which is well localized to the medial joint line owing to its close attachment to the medial collateral ligament. In contrast, pain resulting from lateral meniscal tears is poorly localized. On examination, the sudden inability to extend the knee fully ('locking') strongly suggests a bucket handle type of tear. Other features which may occur include the knee being held in slight flexion, quadriceps wasting in long-standing cases, tenderness over the respective side of the joint (again, better localized in medial meniscal tears), and positive McMurray's and grinding tests.

8 The Trendelenberg sign:
A True
B False
C True
D False
E True

When standing on one leg, the abductors of the hip on the ipsilateral side (gluteus medius, minimus and tensor fasciae latae) contract powerfully to maintain horizontal alignment of the pelvis. This stability is further aided by the integrity of the lever system of the femoral neck and head within the hip joint. Disease processes occurring in these muscles or affecting the lever mechanism may impair the stability of the pelvis and result in it tilting downwards on the opposite side. This is called a positive Trendelenberg sign and causes include:
• Weakness of hip abductors
• Poliomyelitis
• Surgical damage to superior gluteal nerve
• Congenital dislocation of the hip
• Fractured neck of femur
• Shortening of the femoral neck
• Destruction of the femoral head by disease
• Operative removal of head (pseudoarthrosis)
• Severe degree of coxa vara
• Any painful disorder of the hip.

Gluteus medius and minimus are supplied by the superior, not inferior gluteal nerve.

9 Compartment syndrome:
A True
B True
C False
D False
E False

Fractures of the arm or leg result in **bleeding** and **oedema**, two pathological processes which may increase the pressure within an osteofascial compartment. The increased pressure results in reduction in capillary blood flow followed by muscle ischaemia, which causes more oedema and a further rise in intracompartmental pressure. This vicious cycle ends in muscle and nerve necrosis, often within 6 to 12 hours. Nerve is capable of limited regeration, but infarcted muscle does not recover, instead being replaced by inelastic fibrous tissue (Volkmann's ischaemic contracture).

In addition to fractures, compartment syndrome may be caused by a tight plaster cast.

High risk sites for development of compartment syndrome include:
- Around the elbow
- Forearm fractures
- Proximal third of tibia

Clinical features:
- Classic features of ischaemia
- Pain (very severe)
- Paraesthesia
- Pallor
- Paralysis
- Pulselessness (see below)
- Passive hyperextension of fingers or toes; stretching the muscles in the relevant compartment is a sensitive test for muscle ischaemia. Active extension is not helpful as the patient will only move the affected part as far as he can tolerate.

Even if there is no damage to a major vessel, bleeding and oedema can still occur. Thus the presence of a pulse should not deter a diagnosis of compartment syndrome being made. In doubtful cases, intracompartmental pressure can be measured (higher than 40 mmHg supports the diagnosis) but is not usually required for diagnosis. The mainstay of treatment involves prompt decompression of the threatened compartment by open fasciotomy. The wound can then be inspected 5 days later and debridement carried out if necessary, followed by wound suturing, skin grafting or leaving the wound to heal by secondary intention.

10 At the ankle:
A False
B False
C False
D True
E False

Talar shift indicates damage or rupture to the medial ligament of the ankle (deltoid ligament).

At the level of the ankle, flexor hallucis longus (FHL) is lateral to flexor digitorum longus (FDL). The tendon of FHL is crossed in the sole of the foot by the tendons of FDL, thereby restoring FHL to its medial position.

Structures passing posterior to the lateral malleolus (deep to superficial):
- Peroneus longus and brevis
- Sural nerve
- Small saphenous vein

Structures passing posterior to the medial malleolus (deep to superficial):
- Tibialis posterior
- Flexor digitorum longus
- Tibial vein
- Posterior tibial artery
- Tibial nerve
- Flexor hallucis longus

The saphenous nerve and long saphenous vein pass in front of the medial malleolus. The saphenous nerve (branch of the femoral nerve) supplies skin over the medial aspect of the ankle as far forward as the first metatarsophalangeal joint. There are no important neurovascular structures in front of the lateral malleolus.

In normal walking the fibula transmits 25% of body weight through the ankle, almost all of which occurs during heel strike.

11 The following are features of rheumatoid arthritis:
A False
B True
C True
D True
E True

Rheumatoid arthritis is a symmetrical deforming polyarthropathy characterized by chronic inflammation. Approximately 75% will have polyarticular involvement at onset. It most commonly affects the hands and wrists. Cervical spine involvement may cause atlanto-axial subluxation, or rarely spinal cord compression or vertebral artery occlusion. Other joints which may be rarely affected include the temporomandibular joints, and crico-arytenoid joints causing hoarseness of voice, stridor, dyspnoea or dysphagia.

Pleural effusion in rheumatoid arthritis may have a high protein, high white cell count, low glucose, low complement factor C3 and positive rheumatoid factor. The presence of rheumatoid cells, or a positive latex test support the diagnosis.

Radiographic findings include:

Early
• Periarticular osteoporosis
• Erosions

Late
• Loss of joint space
• Bone destruction
• Ankylosis

Laboratory findings:

• Anaemia: normochromic, normocytic
• Raised ESR
• Rheumatoid factor positive in 75–80% of cases, but is also positive in other autoimmune diseases (SLE 40%). False positives may occur in bacterial endocarditis, pulmonary TB, hepatitis and myeloma
• Antinuclear factor positive in 30%
• Synovial fluid: often purulent, of low viscosity, high white cell count, can be sterile on culture

Indications for surgical intervention:
• Carpal tunnel syndrome: if medical management fails
• Ruptured extensor tendons of the hand
• Cord compression: attempt spinal fusion. Note that atlanto-axial subluxation itself does not require any specific surgical treatment
• Baker's cyst: synovectomy if rest and intra-articular steroids fail
• Foot deformities: appropriate shoes, surgical management of hallux valgus
• Painful disease in any joint: for example hip replacement, ankle fusion, excision of ulnar styloid process

12 Osteoarthritis:
A False
B False
C False
D True
E False

Osteoarthritis is defined as a common degenerative condition with a possible inflammatory component. It may be primary or secondary with certain specific subtypes being recognized.

Secondary OA usually involves one joint. Causes include:

• Congenital dislocation of the hip
• Perthe's disease
• Avascular necrosis
• Osteochondritis
• Septic arthritis
• Haemochromatosis
• Gout
• Previous fracture

Primary OA usually involves up to 6 joints, with no definite cause identifiable. Occasionally Heberden's nodes are present.

Primary generalized OA is 10 times more common in females than males. It usually occurs in middle age, with acute episodes of painful, red, warm, tender swollen joints occurring over the course of a few months. The typical chronic picture normally follows. Polyarticular involvement amd the presence of Heberden's nodes are usual.

The use of analgesics is a commonplace first line method of treatment but is not associated with a reduced incidence of the disease.

13 In total hip replacement:
A False
B False
C True
D False
E False

Anterolateral approach: gluteus medius and minimus must be retracted posteriorly to gain access to the joint.

Posterior approach: involves division of the short external rotators of the hip joint (piriformis, obturator internus and the gemelli).

Most hip dislocations occur posteriorly (opposite for shoulder). Thus replacement of a hip by the posterior route will weaken the support on this side of the joint and result in a higher risk of subsequent dislocation than if performed by the anterior approach. The risk of dislocation can be reduced by several intraoperative measures, including using an acetabular cup with a long posterior stem, and ensuring that the cup is positioned with a slight tendency to anteversion. Postoperatively, patients should be encouraged to mobilize early, within 24 to 48 hours under the supervision of a graded physiotherapy programme aimed at restoring muscle strength around the hip. There is no evidence that non-weight bearing for 3–4 days after operation reduces the risk of dislocation.

14 In the foot:
A False
B True
C True
D False
E False

Inversion occurs by any muscle attached to the medial side of the foot. These include tibialis anterior and posterior, assisted by extensor and flexor hallucis longus.
Eversion occurs by any muscle attached to the lateral side of the foot. These include peroneus longus, brevis and tertius. All of these muscles are inserted anterior to the midtarsal joint. In fact the beginning of the movement of either inversion or eversion occurs at the midtarsal joint, followed by movement at the subtalar joints, but most of the full range of these movements occurs at the subtalar joints. The movement of eversion is greatest in dorsiflexion, and is

ultimately limited by tension in the deltoid ligament and tibialis muscles. Inversion is greatest in plantarflexion and is limited by tension in the peroneal muscles and the interosseous talocalcaneal ligament.

The **medial longitudinal arch** consists of calcaneus, talus, navicular, three cuneiform and three metatarsal bones. The stability of the arch is maintained by ligamentous and muscular factors, with bony factors almost negligible. The plantar aponeurosis is the most important ligament, followed by the spring ligament. The most important muscular structures are those that run beneath the arch, namely flexor hallucis longus and to a lesser degree the tendons of flexor digitorum longus to the medial three toes. In contrast, peroneus longus tends to evert and abduct the foot, thereby lowering the medial side of the foot.

The **lateral longitudinal arch** consists of calcaneus, cuboid and the lateral two metatarsal bones. It is much flatter than the medial arch. The plantar aponeurosis is the most important ligamentous stabilizing structure. Its main muscular support comes from peroneus longus and the tendons of flexor digitorum longus to the fourth and fifth toes.

The **transverse arch** is completed as a full arch by that of the other foot. It consists of the bases of the five metatarsal bones, and the adjacent cuboid and cuneiforms. In contrast to the other two arches, some stability is afforded by the bony structure, in particular by the intermediate and lateral cuneiforms which are wedge shaped. The tendon of peroneus longus is the most important factor maintaining the integrity of this arch.

Sensory supply to the skin of the foot:

Deep peroneal nerve   First cleft
Superficial peroneal nerve   Second, third and fourth clefts; medial side of dorsum of great toe
Sural nerve   Lateral side of foot and little toe
Saphenous nerve   Medial side of the foot as

far forward as the first metatarsophalangeal joint
Medial and lateral plantars   Terminal
phalanges and toenails

15 Amputations:
A False
B True
C False
D True
E True

The principles of creating a healthy stump
after an amputation involve healing by first
intention, allowing free mobility of the
stump including joints above it with no
redundant soft tissue, and avoiding the scar
having to transmit pressure. Postoperatively,
exercises to strengthen upper limb muscles
should begin as soon as possible, ideally
before surgery. Exercises to mobilize the
stump can begin within 24 to 48 hours but
weight bearing should not start until day 5
to 6. Assuming a satisfactory stump, a pneu-
matic postamputation mobility aid can be
used to allow mobilization. Prompt fitting of
an artificial limb should be considered.

Inspection of flap bleeding at the time of
surgery is probably better than other means
of determining the likely success of amputation, such as oximetry or Doppler ankle
pressures. Contraindications to a below
knee amputation include osteoarthritis of
the knee, paralysis of the lower limb due to
previous CVA and infection or ischaemia of
the limb requiring a higher amputation.

Complications include:
• Haematoma
• Infection
• Ischaemic necrosis
• Osteomyelitis
• Muscle herniation
• Fixed flexion deformity
• Arteriovenous fistulae and aneurysms
• Causalgia
• Stump neuroma.

16 Congenital dislocation of the hip:
A True
B False
C True
D True
E False

Congenital dislocation of the hip is 7 times
more common in females, occurring more
frequently on the left. Risk factors include a
positive family history, breech presentation,
oligohydramnios and first pregnancy. Ultrasound is useful in demonstrating the position of the hip in infants, and is helpful in
detecting effusions in a limping child to
exclude septic arthritis.

17 Cervical vertebrae:
A False
B False
C False
D True
E True

The **vertebral artery** arises from the first
part of the subclavian artery, on its upper
convexity. It passes up through the pyramidal space to enter the foramina
transversarium of C6 to C2 vertebra. It
ascends vertically anterior to the emerging
spinal nerves, giving a spinal branch into
each intervertebral foramen. Having passed
through the foramina transversarium of the
atlas, it lies in the floor of the suboccipital
triangle before piercing the posterior
atlanto-occipital membrane. It then enters
the skull through the foramen magnum.

The first, second and seventh **cervical
vertebrae** (atlas, axis and vertebra
prominens respectively) are atypical, leaving
four typical cervical vertebrae (3 to 6 inclu-
sive). The **axis** is characterized by the dens
and a large spinous process. The dens is
thought to represent the centrum of the
atlas. It has an articular facet for articulation
with the anterior arch of the atlas, but bears
no weight. The weight of the skull is transmitted through the lateral mass of the atlas
to the superior articular process of the axis,
lateral to the dens.

18 The shoulder:

A True
B False
C True
D False
E False

As with any joint the nerve supply to the shoulder follows **Hilton's Law**: that is, the motor nerve to a muscle tends to give a branch to the joint which is moved by the given muscle (and another branch to the skin over the joint). The shoulder joint thus receives its nerve supply from branches of the axillary, musculocutaneous and suprascapular nerves.

Deltoid is supplied by the axillary nerve (C5, 6), which also supplies teres minor. **Teres major** receives its innervation from the lower subscapular nerve (C5, 6), which also supplies subscapularis (also supplied by the upper subscapular nerve). The **triceps** muscle has three heads. The lateral and medial heads arise from contiguous sides of the back of the humerus with the radial nerve passing in the spiral groove between the two. The long head of triceps is attached to the infraglenoid tubercle. The **rotator cuff muscles** are not all supplied by the posterior cord of the brachial plexus (see Question 1).

The **posterior circumflex humeral artery** passes through the quadrilateral space with the axillary nerve (see Question 1).

19 Disorders of the shoulder:

A True
B True
C False
D True
E False

In the young, **rotator cuff tears** are due to trauma where repair is vigorous and healing rapid. The older patient tends to suffer from degenerative disease in the shoulder resulting in tears that heal more slowly. In general, complete tears are more painful than partial ones. Treatment of complete tears in the initial phase is conservative with heat, exercises and local anaesthetic injec-tions. They should be repaired after 3 weeks in young active individuals but in the elderly in whom tears are commonly pain-less, operation is contraindicated.

The typical clinical picture of **adhesive capsulitis** is that of a patient aged 40–60 with a history of trauma, followed by pain, which gradually increases in severity and then subsides after a few months. At this stage stiffness becomes more severe and may last up to twelve months. The differen-tial diagnosis includes disuse stiffness such as after a stroke or heart attack, and reflex sympathetic dystrophy.

20 In the region of the elbow:

A False
B True
C False
D False
E False

The brachial artery bifurcates at the level of the neck of the radius. Golfer's elbow is medial epicondylitis which is the site of attachment of the common flexor tendon, therefore opposed flexion of the wrist will elicit pain. Opposed extension of the wrist is useful in the diagnosis of lateral epicondylitis or tennis elbow. Fracture of the medial epicondyle should not cause weak-ness of pinch grip between the index finger and thumb because this is action of the first dorsal interosseus muscle supplied by the median nerve. It is the ulnar nerve which is at risk of injury in such fractures.

The capsule of the elbow joint is attached to the annular ligament but not to the radius directly, which allows the head of the radius to pronate and supinate freely.

In elbow arthroscopy, the anteromedial port may damage the medial cutaneous nerve of the forearm, basilic vein and median nerve at a deeper plane. Anterolateral port insertion may damage the lateral cutaneous nerve of the forearm, cephalic vein and posterior interosseus nerve at a deeper level.

21 Metabolic bone disease:
A True
B True
C False
D True
E True

Factors *predisposing* to osteoporosis include old age, immobilization, hypogonadism, Cushing's disease, thyrotoxicosis, hypopituitarism, rheumatoid arthritis, osteogenesis imperfecta, homocystinuria, alcoholism, heparin therapy, smoking and vitamin C deficiency.

Treatment of osteoporosis with bisphosphonates is relatively contraindicated as it reduces bone turnover.

Biochemical markers in osteoporosis tend to be normal whereas osteomalacia is characterized by low calcium, low phosphates and a raised alkaline phosphatase. The low calcium may result in secondary hyperparathyroidism.

22 Radial nerve:
A False
B True
C True
D True
E False

Branches of the radial nerve supply the triceps muscle as they emerge from the axilla, thus fractures of the midshaft of the humerus are unlikely to affect elbow extension. The radial nerve occupies the spiral groove and pierces the lateral intermuscular septum to enter the anterior compartment of the forearm at the level of origin of brachialis.

The sensory branches of the radial nerve given off in the arm include the posterior cutaneous nerve of the arm, lower lateral cutaneous nerve of the arm, and posterior cutaneous nerve of the forearm. In the forearm the posterior interosseus branch has no sensory supply. Radial nerve injuries following fractures of the humerus tend to be axonotmesis with function eventually returning. Exploration may be indicated in an open injury or after 6 weeks if there is no return of function.

23 Dupuytren's disease:
A True
B False
C True
D True
E True

Dupuytren's disease has a prevalence of 5% in the general population and is commonly bilateral. The incidence increases with age and the disease is occasionally associated with a positive family history, in which inheritance is usually autosomal dominant. It can affect the hands or feet, usually the fourth or fifth digits, and is associated with epilepsy, anticonvulsant therapy, heavy manual labour, trauma, diabetes, alcoholic liver disease, Peyronie's disease and AIDS. Pathogenesis is poorly understood but increased xanthine oxidase activity is thought to be a feature. This explains the observation that allopurinol may result in its resolution. Treatment is usually by fasciectomy with Z-plasty of the overlying skin, although late presentation may require joint arthrodesis.

24 Compression of the:
A True
B False
C False
D False
E False

Ulnar nerve lesions at the elbow may be caused by fracture dislocations (especially those resulting in cubitus valgus (Tardy palsy)), osteophytes, Charcot's joints, compression beneath the tendon of flexor carpi ulnaris, student's elbow and leprosy. The ulnar nerve may also be compressed in Guyon's canal at the wrist.

The most reliable test of the **median nerve** is to test the function of abductor pollicis brevis, as the supply to flexor pollicis brevis is subject to more variation than any other muscle in the body.

Injury to the **deep peroneal nerve** would result in inability to dorsiflex the ankle and extend the toes. Damage to the *common* peroneal nerve would in addition cause inability to evert the foot.

25 Carpal tunnel syndrome:

A True

B True

C True

D True

E True

Associations of carpal tunnel syndrome include rheumatoid arthritis, myxoedema, nephrotic syndrome, acromegaly, multiple myeloma, amyloidosis, diabetes mellitus, alcoholism, haemophilia, pregnancy, gout, lipomas, wrist fractures and the menopause.

Weakness of thumb opposition is usually a sign of median nerve impairment due to pressure on the nerve as it passes through the carpal tunnel. It may however rarely be a complication of surgical decompression.

ANSWERS TO EXTENDED MATCHING QUESTIONS

Topic: Paraesthesia

1 A

2 B

3 C
Pain in spondylosis is worse on first getting up in the morning, whereas in carpal tunnel syndrome it is worse at night when the wrist lies in a position of relative flexion.

4 D
A cervical rib may present with a lump in the neck and is usually associated with lower brachial plexus cord lesions.

Topic: Knee pain

1 A
The mechanism of injury is highly suggestive of a meniscal tear, which commonly produces pain highly localized to the medial joint line.

2 B

3 A
Mediolateral movement on knee flexion at 30 degrees is normal, whereas movement on knee extension indicates a collateral ligament injury.

Topic: Bony lesions

1 F

2 D
Ewing's tumour is occasionally associated with adrenal neuroblastoma.

3 C
Osteochondroma occurs as a cartilaginous overgrowth at the edge of the epiphyseal plate. On X-rays it is well defined.

4 G
Hormone replacement therapy is essential for women with early menopause to reduce the risk of osteoporosis.

B: Vascular

1 In the investigation of patients with arterial disease:

A Intravenous digital subtraction angiography may be associated with false aneurysm formation

B Interpretation of duplex ultrasound is made difficult in the presence of atrial fibrillation

C Larger volumes of contrast are required with intra-arterial compared with intravenous digital subtraction angiography

D The diagnosis of vascular disease is more accurately made with post exercise rather than resting Doppler assessment

E The adductor canal is difficult to visualize with duplex ultrasound

2 The femoral triangle:

A The medial boundary is the lateral border of adductor longus

B Contains the profunda femoris artery

C Its superior boundary is the level of termination of the external iliac artery

D The superficial femoral artery is separated from the hip joint by psoas major

E Cannulation of the femoral artery may be complicated by retroperitoneal haemorrhage

3 In a CT scan taken through the upper third of the thigh:

A Psoas major is anterior to the femur

B The sciatic nerve is deep to adductor magnus

C Sartorius is anterior to the femoral vessels

D Profunda femoris passes posteriorly between pectineus and psoas

E Gluteus maximus is not seen

4 Varicose veins:

A Are more common in obese patients

B Are more commonly secondary than familial

C Reduced fibrinolytic activator may be an aetiological factor

D Haemorrhage is a complication

E Not all patients with a past history of lower limb fracture require a duplex scan

5 Thrombophilia may occur in:

A Systemic lupus erythematosus

B Factor V Leiden deficiency

C Increased level of protein C

D Excess antithrombin III

E Pseudogout

6 The subsartorial (adductor) canal:

A Has branches from the anterior division of the obturator nerve in its roof

B Has adductor longus and magnus in its floor

C Contents include the nerve to vastus medialis

D Contents include the saphenous nerve

E Is the commonest site of stenosis of the superficial femoral artery

7 The popliteal fossa:

A Has popliteus muscle in its floor

B The overlying skin is supplied by the posterior cutaneous nerve of the thigh

C The tibial nerve is deep to the popliteal artery

D The roof is pierced by the short saphenous vein

E The sural nerve is between the two heads of gastrocnemius

8 The following are properties of blood flow through a vessel:

A Increased flow is associated with reduced viscosity

B Turbulence is increased in large diameter vessels

C The compliance of the vessel determines the maximum attainable pressure

D As blood flows from a vessel of large diameter to one of small diameter, flow increases whilst resistance decreases

E Apparent viscosity increases non-linearly with haematocrit

9 Pulse pressure is increased:

A In thyrotoxicosis

B With increased arterial compliance

C In mitral valve regurgitation

D In anaemia

E In athletes

10 Collateral circulations:

A Have a higher resistance than in normal vessels

B Compensate for acute arterial occlusions

C Flow is not usually increased during exercise

D Compensate better for superficial femoral than brachial artery occlusions

E Develop as a result of growth of new vessels distal to the stenosis

11 Thrombosis:

A In the axillary vein is commoner on the right

B In the superior vena cava may cause tinnitus

C In the venous system usually consists of fibrin and platelets

D In a proximal leg vein may be an indication for an inferior vena cava filter if the patient also has a peptic ulcer

E Prophylaxis of deep venous thromboses can be achieved by intravenous dextran

12 The following are true about splenectomy:

A All patients require prolonged low dose antibiotic therapy in addition to vaccination

B It is the primary treatment for idiopathic thrombocytopaenia

C Sequelae include a rise in the haemoglobin level

D Left basal atelectasis is common

E Postoperative infection is more common when splenectomy is performed for malignancy than for trauma

13 The spleen:

A Its long axis lies along the ninth rib

B The hilum makes contact with the tail of the pancreas

C Accessory spleens occur in 1% of individuals

D The left kidney indents its medial surface

E Produces IgM antibody

14 The inferior vena cava:

A Has a longer intra-abdominal course than the aorta

B Pierces the central tendon of the diaphragm

C Is formed posterior to the right common iliac artery

D Receives as tributaries the first and second lumbar veins

E Has more valves than the external iliac veins

15 Abdominal aortic aneurysms:

A When infrarenal are associated with suprarenal extension in 10% of cases

B Measuring 5 cm in diameter have a risk of rupture of 5% per year

C Are more commonly saccular than fusiform

D On average expand at the rate of 1 cm per year

E Surgery may be complicated by an extensor plantar response

16 The abdominal aorta:

A Passes behind the medial arcuate ligament of the diaphragm at the level of T12

B Bifurcates at the supracristal plane

C Lies in front of the left lumbar veins

D Normally measures 3 cm in diameter

E The right renal artery is given off at a

level just below that of the inferior mesenteric artery

operative treatment

E   50% require operative intervention

17 A CT scan at the level of L2 would pass through:

A   The origin of the superior mesenteric artery

B   Posterior rami ultimately contributing to the femoral nerve

C   The renal veins joining the inferior vena cava

D   The second part of the duodenum

E   Quadratus lumborum

18 Carotid artery disease:

A   Strokes are more likely to be due to extracranial than intracranial disease

B   Carotid duplex scanning is a good way of assessing the type of carotid plaque that is present

C   A bruit may be absent in a severe stenosis

D   Initial investigation of a patient with a transient ischaemic attack commonly includes a CT scan of the brain

E   Surgery has been shown to be better than medical therapy in the management of asymptomatic patients with stenoses greater than 70%

19 The external carotid artery:

A   Begins at the level of the greater horn of the hyoid bone

B   Is medial to the internal carotid artery at its origin

C   Pulse can be felt by pressing it posteriorly against the transverse process of C6

D   Has the glossopharyngeal nerve between it and the internal carotid artery

E   Surgical approach involves division of investing layer of deep cervical fascia

20 Lymphoedema:

A   Is more likely to occur after radiotherapy than after surgical excision

B   Usually presents as unilateral leg swelling

C   Pitting oedema is usually present early

D   Diuretics can be used as part of non-

21 Arteriovenous fistulae:

A   When secondary to trauma usually form within 36 hours

B   Are characterized clinically by a machinery murmur which is loudest in systole

C   May be associated with a reduced diastolic blood pressure

D   May be associated with increased stroke volume

E   Blood flow distal to the malformation may be reduced

22 Raynaud's phenomenon:

A   Occurs mainly in females under the age of 20

B   Can be treated by a serotonin antagonist

C   Cervical sympathectomy aims to resect the upper part of the stellate ganglion

D   Is associated with hypothyroidism

E   Cervical spondylosis is a cause

23 Cervical rib:

A   Is bilateral in approximately 40% of cases

B   Neurological complications are more common than vascular

C   Treatment includes trapezius strengthening exercises

D   Horner's syndrome is a complication of surgery

E   The C8 nerve root is mainly affected

24 In the root of the neck:

A   Scalenus anterior arises from the anterior tubercles of the typical cervical vertebrae

B   The supreme intercostal vein lies lateral to the first thoracic nerve on the neck of the first rib

C   The scalene tubercle lies posterior to the subclavian artery

D   The phrenic nerve passes anterior to the subclavian vein

E   The vagus nerve passes anterior to the thoracic duct

25 The subclavian artery:

A   Begins at the lateral border of the first rib

B The costocervical trunk arises from the first part

C Blood supply to the first two intercostal spaces posteriorly arises from branches of the thyrocervical trunk

D The subclavian artery and vein are enclosed in a connective tissue sheath derived from the prevertebral fascia

E Becomes the axillary artery at the upper border of teres major

EXTENDED MATCHING QUESTIONS

Topic: Abdominal aortic aneurysm

A Ultrasound of abdomen
B Crossmatch 10 units then immediate surgery
C CT abdomen
D CT chest
E ECG

For each case scenario below, select the most appropriate option from the list above. Each option may be used once, more than once or not at all.

1 A 63-year-old man with a known abdominal aortic aneurysm of 5 cm diameter presents with abdominal and back pain. He has an easily palpable but non-tender expansile abdominal mass and is haemodynamically stable.
2 A 49-year-old smoker is brought into casualty with a history from his relatives of sudden abdominal and chest pain radiating through to the back. He is on medication for severe hypertension. He is pale, with a pulse of 110 per minute and BP 100/60. Examination of his abdomen reveals a tender expansile mass above the umbilicus. Chest X-ray reveals a widened mediastinum of 15 cm.

Topic: Leg ulcers

A Pyoderma gangrenosum
B Neuropathic ulcer
C Ischaemic ulcer
D Venous ulcer
E Squamous cell carcinoma

For each scenario below, select the most appropriate option from the list above. Each option may be used once, more than once or not at all.

1 An ulcer behind the lateral malleolus in a 49-year-old smoker.
2 A 40-year-old diabetic presents with a slowly deepening and painless ulcer over the head of the first metatarsal of her right foot.
3 A 67-year-old man with a long-standing venous ulcer develops pain, with slough in the base. The edge of the ulcer has become raised.
4 A 46-year-old female notices an ulcer over the medial malleolus on the left. She has marked bilateral peripheral oedema.

Topic: Peripheral vascular disease

A Surgical embolectomy
B Femoro-popliteal bypass
C Angioplasty
D Thrombolysis (t-PA)
E Axillo-femoral graft
F Aorto-bifemoral graft

For each scenario below, select the most appropriate treatment option from the list above. Each option may be used once, more than once or not at all.

1 A 76-year-old man presents with rapidly worsening intermittent claudication in his right leg which recently has been extending proximally to involve his thigh and buttock. He has absent pulses below and including the femoral on the right. He is known to have chronic obstructive airways disease for which he receives home nebulizer therapy. An arteriogram demonstrates a diffuse narrowing extending from the origin of his right common iliac artery to the external iliac artery.
2 A 75-year-old man has intermittent claudication in the right leg of 100 metres. He is a smoker, has had 4 myocardial infarctions in the past 5 years, one stroke and is on treatment for hypertension. His ABPI is 0.4 on the right and 0.6 on the left. His arteriogram shows a 2 cm stenosis of 75% in the right common iliac artery with good distal run-off, and a 40% stenosis in the left superficial femoral artery.

3 A 55-year-old man experiences sudden onset left foot pain following a myocardial infarction 2 weeks ago. He normally does not suffer with intermittent claudication. His foot is cold and mottled with no pulses palpable below the knee. He has palpable femoral pulses. An ECG confirms the presence of Q waves.

ANSWERS TO MULTIPLE CHOICE QUESTIONS

1 In the investigation of patients with arterial disease:

A False
B True
C False
D True
E True

Duplex ultrasound combines Doppler and ultrasound, and is a useful although operator dependent non-invasive method of imaging both veins and arteries, particularly the carotid vessels. The adductor canal is the site where the majority of superficial femoral artery occlusions occur and it can be difficult to visualize. It is less accurate if the vessels are heavily calcified, the patient has atrial fibrillation or in proximal vessels where bowel gas can be obscuring.

Intravenous digital subtraction angiography (IV DSA) avoids the need for an arterial puncture but requires large volumes of contrast and depends on a good cardiac output. It is also made more obscure by bowel gas.

Intra-arterial digital subtraction angiography (IA DSA) gives rise to better quality images with less contrast used than IV DSA although is a more invasive procedure. If indicated, angioplasty can also take place on the same occasion. Complications are those of arterial puncture and include false aneurysm formation, dissection, thrombosis, distal embolization and groin haematoma.

2 The femoral triangle:

A False
B False
C True
D False
E True

The femoral triangle is bounded superiorly by the inguinal ligament, laterally by the medial border of sartorius and medially by the *medial* border of adductor longus. The termination of the external iliac artery is at

the level of the inguinal ligament. The floor consists (from lateral to medial) of iliacus, psoas, pectineus, adductor brevis and adductor longus. Its contents include the femoral sheath, itself containing the femoral artery, vein and canal (which itself contains the lymph node of Cloquet), and the femoral nerve (lateral to the artery but outside the femoral sheath). The *common* femoral artery is separated from the capsule of the hip joint by the psoas major muscle; the superficial femoral artery arises at a lower level after the profunda femoris is given off. Complications of femoral artery cannulation are those applicable to puncture of any artery (false aneurysm, dissection, thrombosis, etc.) or those specific to this region which include retroperitoneal haemorrhage and perforation of the gut.

3 In a CT scan taken through the upper third of the thigh:

A True
B False
C True
D False
E False

After passing through the greater sciatic foramen, the sciatic nerve emerges from beneath the lower border of piriformis and is then superficial to the tendons of obturator internus and the gemelli, quadratus femoris and adductor magnus before passing deep to the biceps femoris. At this level, gluteus maximus is seen, the deep part inserting into the gluteal tuberosity of the femur and its more extensive three-quarters inserting into the iliotibial tract with the tensor fascia latae. The profunda femoris artery enters the posterior compartment of the thigh by passing between pectineus and adductor longus. Note how the *adductor longus* muscle lies between the femoral artery (anterior to it) and the profunda femoris artery (posterior to it), and the *adductor brevis* muscle between the anterior division of the obturator nerve (anterior to it) and the posterior division of this nerve (posterior to it).

4 Varicose veins:
A True
B False
C True
D True
E False

Varicose veins affect about 2% of the Western population and are less common in Africans. The majority are *primary*, in particular being associated with increasing age (peak 50–60), female sex, obesity, pregnancy (increased female sex hormones and local pressure effect) and occupations involving prolonged standing. Rarely they may be due to congenital absence of valves or the Klippel-Trenaunay syndrome. *Secondary* varicose veins may be due to obstruction to venous outflow (fibroids, ovarian cyst, pelvic tumours, ascites, iliac vein thrombosis), valve destruction (following deep venous thrombosis) or due to high flow and pressure (arteriovenous fistula). Reduced fibrinolytic activator may be a contributory factor, particularly in familial varicose veins and in leg more than arm veins.

Duplex scans are not needed in all patients with varicose veins as clinical examination is usually sufficient in the majority of cases. However, if there is difficulty in establishing the precise level of reflux, if the veins are recurrent, or if there is a past history of venous thrombosis or lower limb fracture, patients should have a duplex scan to look at the deep and perforating veins in addition to confirming superficial vein incompetence. Note that the reliability of hand held Doppler for establishing saphenopopliteal reflux is not as good as for saphenofemoral reflux. Complications of varicose veins include superficial thrombophlebitis, haemorrhage, lipodermatosclerosis, venous eczema and ulceration.

5 Thrombophilia may occur in:
A True
B False

C False
D False
E False

Causes of **thrombophilia** are *congenital* (activated protein C deficiency, protein S deficiency, antithrombin III deficiency, Factor V Leiden, dysfibrinogenaemia, fibrinolytic defects) and *acquired* (lupus anticoagulant/antiphospholipid syndrome). Factor V Leiden results from a point mutation on the factor V gene giving rise to an abnormal gene product. It is present in 30% of patients with recurrent venous thrombosis. Deficiency of Factor V Leiden is therefore not associated with thrombophilia.

6 The subsartorial (adductor) canal:
A True
B True
C True
D True
E True

The **adductor canal** is an intermuscular cleft distal to the apex of the femoral triangle. The *roof* contains the subsartorial plexus which receives branches from the anterior division of the obturator nerve, saphenous nerve and intermediate cutaneous nerve of the thigh and supplies the overlying fascia lata and skin above the medial aspect of the knee. The *floor* is made up of adductors longus and magnus. The *lateral* border is vastus medialis, and the *anteromedial* border a fibrous sheet deep to sartorius. *Contents* include the superficial femoral artery and vein, the saphenous nerve and the nerve to vastus medialis. This represents the commonest site of stenosis of the superficial femoral artery in the lower limb.

7 The popliteal fossa:
A True
B True
C False
D True
E True

The *roof* of the popliteal fossa is formed by the fascia lata, which is pierced by the short saphenous vein and the posterior femoral cutaneous nerve. The *floor* comprises the popliteal surface of the femur, capsule of the knee joint and the popliteus muscle. The *sural nerve*, a cutaneous branch of the tibial nerve, passes between the two heads of gastrocnemius which comprise the lower boundary of the fossa. In the fossa, the popliteal artery is the deepest of the neurovascular structures, the tibial nerve the most superficial and the popliteal vein in between.

8   The following are properties of blood flow through a vessel:

A   True
B   True
C   False
D   False
E   True

$Q = \Delta P / R$ where Q is flow, ΔP is pressure difference and R is resistance.

Alternatively, $Q = \Delta P \times$ Conductance (given that conductance $= 1/R$).

Poiseuille's law is embodied in the formula $R = 8\eta l / \pi r^4$ where h is viscosity, l is length and r is the radius of the vessel.

Thus: $Q = (\Delta P \times \pi r^4)/8\eta l$

From this it can be seen that viscosity (η) varies inversely with flow (Q) and proportionately with vessel diameter ($r \times 2$). *Apparent viscosity* describes the value of blood viscosity relative to that of plasma. In small vessels, axial flow of red blood cells occurs centrally with plasma flow peripherally, which enables faster flow of cells and therefore a lower apparent viscosity. Apparent viscosity increases with increasing haematocrit but the relationship is non-linear.

As the radius of a vessel decreases, flow does not necessarily decrease. This is because $Q =$ velocity $\times$ cross sectional area. The velocity of flow increases with reduced radius of the vessel whilst the viscosity decreases (see above), thereby helping the flow to increase to or beyond normal. However, resistance will also increase with reduced radius, thus limiting the overall increase in flow.

The *compliance* of a vessel reflects the change in volume for a given change in pressure. It is less with advancing age and at the extremes of blood pressure. When cardiac output increases, compliance affects the rate of rise of pressure but not the maximum pressure attained. *Turbulence* is given by the Reynold's number N_R, which is increased in large diameter vessels with high velocity and low viscosity.

9   Pulse pressure is increased:

A   True
B   False
C   False
D   True
E   True

The pulse pressure equals the difference between systolic and diastolic pressure. Factors which affect it are those which contribute to blood pressure, i.e. cardiac output and total peripheral resistance. Cardiac output is affected by stroke volume and heart rate, whilst peripheral resistance by arterial compliance. Thus in athletes pulse pressure will be increased on account of the increased stroke volume despite the possibly reduced heart rate. Pulse pressure will also be raised in thyrotoxicosis or anaemia where heart rate is raised. Patients with aortic but not mitral valve regurgitation have a greater stroke volume resulting from an increased end diastolic volume. This gives rise to a greatly increased pulse pressure and the clinical feature of waterhammer pulse.

If the compliance is reduced, the systolic pressure increases and the diastolic pressure reduces such that the pulse pressure is in fact higher.

10 Collateral circulations:
A True
B False
C True
D False
E False

Collateral channels develop from the enlargement of existing vessels, as a result of an increased amount of blood being required to pass through them due to a stenosis. As these channels take time to develop fully, chronic occlusions are tolerated better than acute occlusions. Occlusion of iliac and femoral arteries are also better tolerated by the development of collaterals than brachial occlusions. The resistance is almost always higher in collateral than normal vessels. Flow through these channels is also not usually increased during exercise as the resistance vessels are usually dilated maximally.

11 Thrombosis:
A True
B True
C False
D True
E False

Arterial thrombi most often form in areas of atherosclerotic damage. They develop alternating layers of fibrin and aggregated platelets (lines of Zahn) which macroscopically gives them a white appearance. Venous thrombi form in areas of blood stasis and as a result have a greater concentration of red blood cells (red thrombus). They are less likely to have lines of Zahn. Intravenous dextrans reduces the risk of pulmonary embolism but not of deep venous thrombosis. Indications for an inferior vena cava filter in a proximal deep venous thrombosis include an acute bleeding duodenal ulcer, pregnancy or a recent CVA as in these circumstances thrombolytic therapy is relatively or absolutely contraindicated. Axillary vein thrombosis is in fact more common on the right than the left. Superior vena cava thrombosis may give rise to tinnitus, epistaxis or cough.

12 The following are true about splenectomy:
A False
B True
C True
D True
E True

Splenectomy is indicated in trauma either following an accident or iatrogenic injury (such as following mobilization of the splenic flexure), to reduce the thrombocytopenia in idiopathic thrombocytopenic purpura or hypersplenism, removal with the stomach as part of a radical gastrectomy, removal as part of a staging procedure in Hodgkin's lymphoma or for portal hypertension (in association with shunt surgery). **Postoperative complications** particularly related to this operation include haemorrhage, gastric dilatation, left basal atelectasis with or without a pleural effusion, damage to the tail of the pancreas and various haematological sequelae including rise in white cell, platelet, and haemoglobin count. The blood volume may also fall, and this in combination with thrombocythaemia predisposes to thrombosis. **Post-splenectomy infection** is typically by encapsulated bacteria in particular *Streptococcus pneumoniae, Neisseria meningitidis* and *Haemophilus influenzae*. The risk is higher in children than in adults, and when splenectomy is performed for malignancy than for trauma. Children should receive pneumococcal vaccine (and HIB/meningo- coccal vaccines if available) and antibiotic prophylaxis until 18 years of age. The vaccines may need to be repeated to remain effective in the long term. Adults should receive pneumococcal vaccine particularly prior to splenectomy being performed for haematological disorders or malignancy. There is no place for prophylactic antibiotics for life unless it is the wish of the patient.

13 The spleen:
A False
B True

C   False
D   True
E   True

The spleen measures $25 \times 75 \times 130$ mm (1×3 $\times 5$ inches). It lies between the ninth and eleventh ribs with its long axis along the line of the tenth. It is not essential for life but has several functions, including immunoglobulin production (mainly IgM), destruction of abnormally shaped red cells, phagocytosis of foreign substances, as a platelet reservoir and red cell production *in utero*. The hilum comes into contact with the tail of the pancreas within the lienorenal ligament, and in addition comprises the gastrosplenic ligament and lesser sac. The medial surface of the spleen is indented by the left kidney, stomach and splenic flexure of colon. The spleen develops in the dorsal mesogastrium from condensations of mesenchyme which normally aggregate into a single mass. Accessory spleens arise from the lack of fusion of these condensations and occur in 10% of individuals.

14 The inferior vena cava:
A   True
B   True
C   True
D   False
E   False

The inferior vena cava (IVC) commences at the level of L5 and leaves the abdomen by piercing the central tendon of the diaphragm to pass through the caval opening at T8. In contrast the **aorta** enters the abdomen at the level of T12 and bifurcates into the common iliac arteries at L4. Thus the IVC has a longer intra-abdominal course. The IVC is formed behind the right common iliac artery (and is thus initially partly behind the aorta) and ascends to lie in front and to the right of the aorta by the level of the renal arteries. The right sympathetic trunk is therefore posterior to the IVC. The third and fourth lumbar veins drain directly into the IVC. The first and second lumbar veins drain into the ascending

lumbar vein which joins the subcostal vein to form the azygos and hemiazygos veins. The inferior vena cava and common iliac veins usually have no valves, with more distal veins having progressively more and more valves.

15 Abdominal aortic aneurysms:
A   False
B   True
C   False
D   False
E   True

An aneurysm is a localized fixed dilatation of a blood vessel or of the heart. Of the abdominal aorta, 95% are due to atherosclerosis and 95% infrarenal although 2% are associated with suprarenal extension. They are usually fusiform in shape. On average they grow at the rate of 0.5 cm per year. From Laplace's relationship in which wall tension increases in proportion to the fourth power of the radius, a small increase in aneurysm size markedly increases the tension in the wall and thus its propensity to rupture. Thus a 5 cm aneurysm has a 5% risk, 5.5 cm 10–15% and 7 cm 75% risk of rupture per year. A small proportion of patients with ruptured aneurysms will survive, thus the corresponding figures for mortality at one year are slightly lower. The operative mortality for an elective repair is between 2 and 10%. Thus a 5 cm aneurysm has a lower mortality at 1 year if left alone than if it were operated on, whereas with a 5.5 cm aneurysm the figures are more in balance. A decision to operate will also rest on other factors including the rate of expansion (if significantly greater than 1 cm per year, elective repair may be considered sooner), type of aneurysm (saccular aneurysms are more likely to rupture and thus warrant earlier surgery) and patient fitness. Complications of surgery are mainly respiratory (atelectasis, consolidation) but also include haemorrhage, renal failure, colonic ischaemia, impotence, graft infection, aortoduodenal fistula and spinal cord ischaemia leading to paraplegia.

16 The abdominal aorta:

A False
B True
C True
D True
E False

The aorta enters the abdominal cavity by passing between the crura of the diaphragm and behind the median arcuate ligament at the level of T12. It inclines gently to the left as it descends before bifurcating at the level of L4 (denoted in surface anatomy by the supracristal plane, a line joining the highest points of the iliac crests). It is normally 2 cm in diameter. It lies anterior to the left lumbar veins and left sympathetic trunk. The coeliac trunk arises at the level of T12, and the superior mesenteric artery at L1, between which are found the pancreas and splenic vein. The inferior mesenteric artery arises at the level of L3, and between this and the superior mesenteric artery are found the third part of the duodenum and left renal vein. The renal arteries arise at the level of L2.

17 A CT scan at the level of L2 would pass through:

A False
B True
C True
D True
E True

A line passing through L2 will pass below the origin of the superior mesenteric artery which arises at the level of L1. The second and fourth parts of the duodenum are also found at this level. The roots of the femoral nerve arise from the posterior primary rami of L2 and L3; the anterior rami of L2 and L3 ultimately form the obturator nerve. The renal veins join the vena cava at the level of L2. Quadratus lumborum arises from the transverse process of L5 and iliac crest, and fibres pass upwards lateral to psoas to the transverse processes of the upper 4 lumbar vertebrae and medial half of the twelfth rib.

18 Carotid artery disease:

A False
B True
C True
D True
E False

Atherosclerosis is common at the bifurcation of the common carotid artery where initially it causes asymptomatic stenoses of the origins of the internal and external carotid arteries. A patient with an asymptomatic stenosis of 50% or more has a risk of around 2% per year of developing a stroke. Following a stroke or transient ischaemic attack (TIA), the risk of developing a subsequent stroke is about 10% in the first year then 5% per year. About 30% of strokes arise secondary to extracranial carotid disease. Bruits are an unreliable guide to the presence or severity of carotid stenoses. They may be absent in the most severe stenoses where blood cannot get through at all, or may be transmitted sounds from the heart in the absence of carotid disease. Duplex imaging is capable of assessing plaque morphology but is not reliable at visualizing the vertebral system and may be obscured by significant vessel calcification. A CT scan is a useful investigation in a patient who has had a TIA as it will help initially to exclude a haemorrhagic component and also subsequently serves to exclude intracranial lesions that might mimic ischaemic episodes (e.g. tumours). The **European Carotid Surgery Trial (ECST)** and the **North American Symptomatic Carotid Endarterectomy Trial (NASCET)** both concluded that in patients who had experienced a TIA, non-disabling stroke or retinal infarct within the preceding 4–6 months, carotid endarterectomy with medical therapy (usually aspirin) resulted in a lower subsequent rate of re-infarct for severe (70–99%) stenoses than in patients who received medical therapy alone. The ECST also found that there was no benefit gained in terms of stroke prevention from endarterectomy for patients with mild (<30%) or moderate (30–69%) symptomatic stenoses. Thus, as only symptomatic patients with stenoses greater than 70% require surgery, asymptomatic patients do not require surgery as long as their stenoses are less than 70%. There is no consensus yet as to whether asymptomatic patients with >70% stenoses benefit from surgery.

19 The external carotid artery:
A True
B True
C False
D True
E True

The origin of the **external carotid artery** is said to be at the upper border of the thyroid cartilage (C4) although it is commonly higher, at the level of the greater horn of the hyoid bone (C3). At this point it is medial to the internal carotid artery but as they ascend it gradually drifts to assume a more lateral position. It passes through the parotid gland and is separated from the internal carotid artery by the deep part of the gland, stylopharyngeus, glossopharyngeal nerve and pharyngeal branch of the vagus. The carotid pulse involves compression of the *common* carotid artery posteriorly against the transverse process of C6 vertebrae (carotid tubercle of Chassaignac). The artery is enclosed within the carotid sheath which is free to glide over the prevertebral fascia posteriorly, but anteriorly is loosely attached to the deep surface of sternocleidomastoid. Thus surgical approach of the artery involves incision of the investing layer of deep cervical fascia medial to sternocleidomastoid, followed by exposure of the carotid sheath.

20 Lymphoedema:
A True
B True
C True
D False
E False

Lymphoedema is tissue fluid accumulation as a result of an abnormality of the lymphatic system. The legs are affected in

80% of cases. Lymphoedema *secondary* to a definable cause is more common than *primary* lymphoedema. Causes include infection in particular filariasis (*Wuchereria bancrofti*), radiotherapy, surgical excision, chronic inflammation (rheumatoid arthritis) and artefactual. Radiotherapy is more likely to give rise to lymphoedema than surgical excision alone. It usually presents as unilateral leg swelling although the commonest cause of unilateral ankle oedema is long-standing venous disease. In the early stages the oedema usually pits readily, but with time chronic fibrosis leads to the characteristic non-pitting oedema. Ninety per cent respond to conservative and medical treatment. This involves elevation which reduces intravascular pressure, grade III compression stockings (40 mmHg compression or more) which increase extravascular hydrostatic pressure, and massage which aids flow of fluid proximally. Diuretics are generally unhelpful. Surgery is only required in the 10% of patients who do not respond to the above measures.

21 Arteriovenous fistulae:
A False
B True
C True
D True
E True

Arteriovenous fistulae (AVF) may be traumatic (either spontaneous or iatrogenic injury following arterial puncture) or surgically fashioned (such as a Cimino fistula for haemodialysis). They take several days to form when due to trauma. Clinically they have a palpable thrill and an audible continuous machinery murmur which is loudest in systole and disappears when the fistula is occluded. *Branham's test* may be used to assess the degree to which the AVF is affecting the cardiac output. In this test the pulse rate is recorded for one minute before the fistula is occluded. The pulse is then measured again. If there is a marked fall in pulse rate in the second reading, this is indicative of a sizeable left to right shunt.

Other haemodynamic effects of AVF's include a reduced systolic and diastolic blood pressure, increased heart rate and jugular venous pressure and reduced arterial blood flow distal to the AVF.

22 Raynaud's phenomenon:
A True
B True
C False
D False
E True

Raynaud's disease is by definition idiopathic. **Raynaud's phenomenon** describes the intermittent constriction of digital vessels on exposure to cold giving rise to the typical colour change from white to blue to red. It occurs most commonly in females below the age of 20. Causes include collagen vascular diseases (e.g. SLE, scleroderma), cervical rib, cervical spondylosis, Buerger's disease, syringomyelia, increased plasma viscosity (e.g. cryoglobulinaemia), drugs (e.g. β-blockers) and vibrating tools. Medical treatment includes the calcium channel antagonist nifedipine, serotonin antagonists, prostaglandins such as PGI_2 and transdermal glyceryltrinitrate. Surgical therapy may involve resection of a cervical rib, or cervical sympathectomy which aims to resect the upper thoracic sympathetic ganglion whilst preserving the upper part of the stellate ganglion.

23 Cervical rib:
A False
B True
C True
D True
E False

Cervical ribs are bilateral in 70% of cases. Neurological complications are twenty times more common than vascular ones and predominantly affect the T1 nerve root. They may present with a mass in the neck, distal embolization and neck bruit secondary to post-stenotic arterial dilatation, distal ischaemia due to arterial spasm, Horner's syndrome, Raynaud's phenomenon, or paraesthesiae, weakness or numbness in the hand or arm suggestive of T1 root compression. Management involves improving posture and trapezius strengthening exercises. Surgical decompression is reserved for resistant cases as it does not always relieve symptoms and is associated with complications including Horner's syndrome due to injury to the stellate ganglion, pneumothorax and brachial plexus injury.

24 In the root of the neck:
A True
B False
C False
D False
E True

Four structures cross the neck of the first rib; from medial to lateral they are the sympathetic chain, the supreme intercostal vein and artery and the T1 nerve root. Scalenus anterior arises from the anterior tubercles of the typical cervical vertebrae. The *scalene tubercle* into which the scalenus anterior muscle inserts is on the inner border and upper surface of the first rib. The subclavian artery is posterior to this, being divided into its three parts by scalenus anterior, and the subclavian vein is anterior. The *phrenic nerve* passes down on the anterior surface of scalenus anterior beneath the prevertebral fascia. It crosses anterior to the subclavian artery but posterior to the subclavian vein. On the left the *vagus nerve* passes anterior to the thoracic duct.

25 The subclavian artery:
A False
B False
C False
D False
E False

The **right subclavian artery** originates as one of the two terminal branches of the brachiocephalic artery behind the right sternoclavicular joint. The **left subclavian artery** arises directly from the arch of the aorta and ascends with the left common carotid artery before turning laterally at the left sternoclavicular joint. It is divided into three parts by the *scalenus anterior* muscle (see Q24 for origin and insertion). The *first* part (medial to scalenus anterior) has *three* branches, the vertebral artery, the internal thoracic artery and the thyrocervical trunk which gives off the transverse cervical, suprascapular and inferior thyroid arteries. The *second* part lies behind scalenus anterior and has *one* branch, the costocervical trunk which gives off the superior intercostal artery (supplying blood to the first two intercostal spaces posteriorly) and deep cervical artery. The *third* part (lateral to scalenus anterior) has *no* branches. From the lateral border of scalenus anterior the trunks of the brachial plexus and the subclavian artery are enclosed in a continuation of prevertebral fascia called the *axillary sheath*. The axillary and subclavian veins are not enclosed in this sheath, which enables them to expand in response to increased blood flow. The subclavian artery becomes the axillary artery at the outer border of the first rib (the axillary artery becomes the brachial artery at the lower border of teres major).

Topic: Abdominal aortic aneurysm

1 C

This man does not require emergency surgery as his aneurysm is non-tender and he is haemodynamically stable. However in view of his back pain his aneurysm needs further assessment by investigation. In this circumstance a CT scan is preferable to an ultrasound as it is better at identifying small leaks from the aorta, and also for looking at suprarenal extension. Ultrasound is adequate for outpatient assessment of aneurysm size.

2 D

The history and examination suggest strongly that this man has an abdominal aortic aneurysm (AAA) which is probably leaking. The chest X-ray also suggests that he may also have pathology in his thoracic aorta, either dissection or an aneurysm which may be separate from or a continuation of his AAA. In this case surgery cannot proceed for his AAA until a CT scan of his chest has been performed. If the X-ray findings are confirmed, this will change the nature of any surgery that this man may receive – operative repair of both thoracic and abdominal pathologies may proceed or may be cancelled if the overall operative mortality is deemed to be too high.

Topic: Leg ulcers

1 C

2 B

3 E

This is known as a Marjolin's ulcer.

4 D

Topic: Peripheral vascular disease

1 E

This gentleman needs a revascularization procedure. Although an aorto-femoral graft ought to be technically feasible, abdominal surgery would be unadvisable in this man who has significant co-morbidity. An axillo-femoral graft is a less invasive surgical option although patency rates are not as good as for aorto-femoral grafts.

2 C

This man has a short segment stenosis which is amenable to angioplasty. The left lesion need not be treated as this side is currently asymptomatic.

3 A

This man has suffered an acute thromboembolic event almost certainly secondary to his MI. As he is now 2 weeks from the presumed start of the embolic episode, surgical embolectomy is a better option than thrombolysis.

C: Head and Neck

1 Congenital hypertrophic pyloric stenosis:

A Has an incidence similar to that of intussusception

B Recurs in 3% after treatment

C Barium meal is commonly used in demonstrating the pyloric tumour

D Hyponatraemia may occur

E Presents with bile-stained vomiting

2 Causes of jaundice in infants include:

A Choledochal cyst

B Galactosaemia

C Gilbert's syndrome

D Diabetes

E Biliary atresia

3 Tonsillitis:

A Is most commonly caused by the bacteria *S. pneumoniae* and *H. influenzae*

B Of viral aetiology usually results in more profound tonsillar swelling than that of bacterial aetiology

C Otalgia is due to referred pain from the vagus nerve to the tympanic plexus

D Emergency surgery is mandatory for secondary haemorrhage occurring 7 days post-tonsillectomy

E Complicated by retropharyngeal abscess should be treated by tonsillectomy

4 Regarding laryngeal pathology:

A Vocal cord nodules are more common in children than adults

B Vocal cord polyps usually occur one-third of the way along the vocal cords from the anterior commissure

C Granulomas associated with endotracheal intubation are usually located midway along the vocal cords

D External laryngocoeles extend beyond the thyrohyoid membrane

E Alcohol is an independent risk factor for chronic laryngitis

5 Laryngeal nerve palsy:

A Of the superior laryngeal nerve cause reduction of cord adduction

B Of the recurrent laryngeal nerve may cause loss of sensation in the supraglottis

C Patients with unilateral palsy of the recurrent laryngeal nerve may not have hoarseness

D Treatment by Teflon® injection should not be delayed more than 6 to 9 months from diagnosis

E 40% of cases of recurrent laryngeal nerve palsy are idiopathic

6 The normal full term infant:

A Weighing 3 kg has an energy requirement of about 1674 J (400 calories) per day

B Has a higher percentage of intracellular water than in a 70 kg adult

C Has a blood volume of approximately 250 mL

D Is unable to conserve urinary sodium

E Increases his respiratory rate rather than tidal volume when respiratory function needs to be increased

7 The facial nerve:

A Occupies the antero-superior quadrant of the internal acoustic meatus

B Motor fibres synapse in the geniculate ganglion

C Supplies buccinator

D A lower motor neurone palsy may cause ptosis

E Has a sensory supply to the tympanic membrane

8 Temporal lobe abscesses:

A Are most commonly caused by middle ear infections

B May cause nystagmus

C Cause diplopia in 30% of cases

D Characteristically cause a lower quadrantic homonymous hemianopia

E May cause hearing loss

9 Phaeochromocytomas:

A A high proportion of adrenaline is said to favour an adrenal source

B Are more commonly extra-adrenal in children

C Preoperative α-blockade should be started before β-blockade

D May cause postural hypotension

E Produce noradrenaline as the predominant catecholamine

10 Umbilical herniae:

A In neonates require urgent surgery due to the risk of strangulation

B Preoperative weight reduction reduces mortality in elective cases

C Cause pain due to trapping of extraperitoneal fat

D In adults are uncommon before the age of 40

E Faecal fistula is a recognized complication

11 The following are true about the submandibular salivary gland:

A In excision of the gland, the hypoglossal nerve is seen crossing the submandibular duct

B It overlaps the insertion of the medial pterygoid muscle

C Adenolymphomas typically occur in elderly patients

D The superficial part extends between hyoglossus and mylohyoid

E It may be involved in mumps

12 The lingual artery:

A Overlies the hypoglossal nerve

B Passes deep to hyoglossus

C Arises from the anterior aspect of the external carotid artery

D Supplies the submandibular salivary gland

E Supplies the anterior two-thirds but not the posterior one-third of the tongue

13 The following are true about the parotid gland:

A Within the gland the facial nerve is deep to the external carotid artery

B Stensen's duct pierces buccinator at the level of the second upper molar tooth

C Preauricular lymph nodes are commonly found within its substance

D Parotid calculi typically give rise to episodes of pain which are of longer duration than episodes of pain due to submandibular calculi

E As a complication of parotidectomy, Frey's syndrome typically occurs at around 3 months postoperatively

14 Nerves supplying sensation to the external auditory meatus include:

A Auriculotemporal

B Glossopharyngeal

C Vagus

D Facial

E Great auricular

15 The lateral pterygoid muscle:

A Is attached to the greater wing of the sphenoid bone

B Inserts into the articular disc of the temporomandibular joint

C Lies lateral to the mandibular nerve

D Contributes to the protrusion of the mandible

E Is supplied by the lingual nerve

16 Concerning thyroidectomy:

A When performed for Graves' disease, carbimazole should be continued for 2 days postoperatively

B Preoperative use of β-blockers helps to reduce peripheral conversion of T_4 to T_3

C Postoperative hypocalcaemia may be due to reversal of osteoporosis

D Sternohyoid and sternothyroid are usually divided to provide good exposure

E The superior thyroid artery is usually ligated as close to the upper pole of the thyroid as possible

17 The following are true about the adrenal glands:

A The right adrenal is overlapped by the inferior vena cava

B The left adrenal is pyramidal in shape

C The blood supply in part derives from the inferior phrenic artery

D The right adrenal vein is shorter than the left

E The zona glomerulosa produces cortisol

18 The Eustachian tube:

A Is shorter and more horizontal in children than adults

B Its cartilaginous part opens into the nasopharynx

C Its bony part perforates the petrous part of the temporal bone

D Is lined by respiratory epithelium along its entire length

E Is opened by contraction of salpingopharyngeus

19 The posterior triangle of the neck:

A Contains the axillary vein

B In the roof the accessory nerve is embedded within the investing layer of deep cervical fascia

C On the floor the accessory nerve lies upon levator scapulae

D The external jugular vein pierces the roof to enter the triangle

E Contains the transverse cervical artery

20 Thyroglossal cysts:

A Are situated in the midline in 90% of cases

B Are more common in males

C Occur most commonly in the second decade

D Surgery involves removal of part of the hyoid bone

E Originate from between the filiform and vallate papillae of the tongue

21 There is a higher chance of a solitary thyroid nodule being malignant in:

A Males than females

B Patients over 40 years of age

C The presence of recurrent laryngeal nerve palsy

D Thyrotoxic patients

E The presence of a multinodular goitre

22 Hirschsprung's disease:

A Is more common in males

B Is associated with Down's syndrome in 10% of cases

C The diagnosis is confirmed by the presence of nerve trunks demonstrated on rectal mucosal biopsy

D Excision of the affected segment is the treatment of first choice

E Is the commonest cause of intestinal obstruction in the newborn

23 Concerning radioiodide therapy:

A It is indicated in the treatment of thyroid cancer with extracapsular disease

B Thyroxine replacement should not be stopped until the therapy is started

C The incidence of hypothyroidism is similar to that after thyroidectomy

D It shows a good response in the treatment of medullary carcinoma of the thyroid

E Hyperparathyroidism is a recognized complication

24 The following relate to the thyroid gland:

A The right recurrent laryngeal nerve is more likely to lie behind than in front of the inferior thyroid artery

B The isthmus lies anterior to the cricopharyngeal sphincter

C Primary abnormality of TSH production is a common cause of hypothyroidism

D T_3 is 5 times more physiologically active than T_4

E The majority of T_3 and T_4 are bound to albumin

25 Hypercalcaemia:

A Commonly occurs in disseminated carcinoma of the prostate

B May cause subperiosteal erosions in the phalanges

C May be treated with intravenous saline and thiazide diuretics

D Due to malignancy is often associated with a hypochloraemic metabolic alkalosis

E Due to primary hyperparathyroidism is more likely to be due to hyperplasia than adenoma

Topic: Adrenal hyperfunction

A Cushing's disease
B Phaeochromocytoma
C Pseudo-Cushing's syndrome
D Adrenal adenoma
E Ectopic ACTH production

For each of the scenarios below, select the single most likely diagnosis from the list of options above. Each option may be used once, more than once or not at all.

1 A 35-year-old male presents with proximal muscle weakness, truncal obesity and hypertension. There is no suppression with the overnight dexamethasone suppression test but there is suppression with the high dose dexamethasone suppression test. Plasma ACTH is raised.
2 A 45-year-old male presents with proximal muscle weakness, truncal obesity and hypertension. There is no suppression with either the overnight or the high dose dexamethasone suppression test. Plasma ACTH is raised.
3 A 22-year-old female presents with proximal muscle weakness, truncal obesity and hypertension. There is no suppression with the overnight dexamethasone suppression test but there is suppression with the 48 hour low dose dexamethasone suppression test.
4 Assay of CRF from the petrosal sinus may help distinguish Cushing's disease from this condition.

Topic: Abdominal pain in children

A Infantile pyloric stenosis
B Intussusception
C Meconium ileus
D Hirschsprung's disease
E Appendicitis
F Meckel's diverticulum

For each of the patients below, select the single most likely diagnosis from the list of options above. Each option may be used once, more than once or not at all.

1 A 6-month-old boy presents with abdominal pain and a mass palpable in the periumbilical region. This is followed by passage of blood in the stool.
2 A 4-week-old girl presents with weight loss and vomiting. Her parents have been feeding her more frequently than normal.
3 A 4-year-old boy presents with right iliac fossa pain and a hypochromic microcytic anaemia.

Topic: Inguino-scrotal problems

A Testicular cancer
B Hydrocele
C Torsion of the Hydatid of Morgagni
D Epididymal cyst
E Retractile testis
F Maldescended testis

For each of the patients below, select the single most likely diagnosis from the list of options above. Each option may be used once, more than once or not at all.

1 An 18-year-old man presents with a testicular lump which does not transilluminate. His testicle cannot be distinguished from the lump.
2 A 13-year-old boy presents with testicular pain. Examination reveals a small lump at the upper pole with a slight blue discolouration.
3 A 6-month-old boy presents with a lump in the left inguinal region which can only be milked as far as the fundus of the scrotum. The size is similar to that of a normal testis.

ANSWERS TO MULTIPLE CHOICE QUESTIONS

1 Congenital hypertrophic pyloric stenosis:

A True
B False
C False
D True
E False

The incidence of congenital hypertrophic pyloric stenosis (CHPS) and that of intususseption are similar, approximating to 1 in 250. CHPS presents with projectile vomiting which is not bile stained. It tends not to recur after treatment by Ramstedt's pyloromyotomy whereas intussusception recurs in 3%. Ultrasound is generally the preferred investigation in the confirmation of visible peristalsis although barium meal may be employed in difficult cases. As a result of loss of acid from the stomach, renal compensation occurs to preserve H^+ ions which takes place at the expense of sodium loss.

2 Causes of jaundice in infants include:

A True
B True
C False
D True
E True

Transient early jaundice is a common finding in normal neonates during the first 24 to 48 hours. Bilirubin is mainly unconjugated (i.e. lipid soluble and albumin bound). Surgical causes of jaundice in infants include biliary atresia and choledochal cyst. Other non-surgical causes include haemolytic disease of the newborn, infection, maternal diabetes, galactosaemia and hypothyroidism.

3 Tonsillitis:

A False
B True
C False
D False
E False

The incidence of tonsillitis has a peak at 5 to 7 years of age and another smaller peak in adolescence. Common bacterial causative organisms include β-haemolytic streptococci and *S. faecalis*. Viral organisms include Epstein–Barr virus, adenovirus, rhinovirus and HIV. Tonsillar swelling tends to be more severe in viral rather than bacterial aetiology, increasing the likelihood of obstructive symptoms. Otalgia is due to referred pain along Jacobsen's nerve, which is the tympanic branch of the glossopharyngeal nerve.

Complications of tonsillitis include obstruction to breathing, dysphagia, sturtor (voice affected due to palatal splinting), parapharyngeal abscess formation (risk to carotid structures) or retropharyngeal abscess (or quinsy). The latter is treated by lancing although milder cases may respond to parenteral antibiotics.

Haemorrhage is the main complication of tonsillectomy. When primary it is usually due to inadequate control of bleeding at operation or due to a slipped ligature, and may require return to theatre for definitive control. When secondary it is usually due to infection which is managed initially by appropriate resuscitation and local control of bleeding such as by adrenaline soaked gauze applied firmly to the fauces, followed by parenteral antibiotics and intravenous fluids. Surgery is rarely required in this case.

4 Regarding laryngeal pathology:

A True
B False
C False
D True
E True

Vocal cord *nodules* are more common in children than adults and in females than males. They usually occur one-third of the way along from the anterior commissure of the larynx, i.e. one-half of the way along the true vocal cords. Vocal cord *polyps* are more common in adults than children and in males than females. They may occur anywhere on the vocal cords. **Granulomas** associated with endotracheal intubation are classically found in a posterior position on the vocal cords. **Laryngoceles** are air-filled sacs which develop secondary to increased pressure within the saccule. When they spread to the false cords, they are *internal*; when they protrude through the thyrohyoid membrane, they are *external*. Internal ones can be excised from the false cords via laryngoscopy; external ones are excised through a neck incision.

5 Laryngeal nerve palsy:

A True
B False
C True
D False
E True

The **superior laryngeal nerve** gives rise to a large internal laryngeal nerve which pierces the thyrohyoid membrane to provide sensation to the larynx above the vocal cords, and a small external laryngeal nerve which passes in close proximity to the superior laryngeal vessels outside the larynx to supply the cricothyroid muscle. This muscle lengthens and adducts the true vocal cords; these actions are lost if the superior laryngeal nerve is injured, giving rise to a voice which cannot attain the highest of pitches.

The **recurrent laryngeal nerve** passes upwards under the lower border of the inferior constrictor behind the cricothyroid joint to supply all of the intrinsic muscles of the larynx except cricothyroid, together with providing sensation to the larynx below the vocal cords. In 40% of cases of recurrent laryngeal nerve palsy, no cause is identified. Unilateral paralysis will initially result in a hoarse and breathy voice as the cord adopts the paramedian position, but compensation from the contralateral vocal cord occurs (due to the action of interarytenoid) causing the voice to return to normal. Treatment is observation for 6 to 9 months as recovery can spontaneously occur. If there is no improvement in voice by this time, Teflon®

injection lateral to the vocalis muscle can be tried. Bilateral paralysis is usually secondary to thyroidectomy; the cords may be either in the abducted or adducted position, and care must be taken as an urgent tracheostomy may be required.

6 The normal full term infant:

A False
B True
C True
D True
E True

A normal full term infant requires about 420 J (or 100 calories) per kilogram per 24 hours for maintenance and growth. Average blood volume is between 80 to 100 mL per kilogram. When the infant becomes stressed, minute volume (which equals the product of tidal volume and the number of breaths in 1 minute) increases. The tidal volume remains relatively constant, thus the respiratory rate must be increased above its normal level of 35 breaths per minute. Intracellular water comprises 35% total body water in neonates and 40% in adults. Extracellular water comprises 40% total body water in neonates and 20% in adults. In addition total body water comprises 80% of the weight of a neonate compared with 65% of an adult's body weight.

7 The facial nerve:

A True
B False
C True
D False
E True

The **facial nerve** exits the cerebellopontine angle as two separate roots: the *motor root* (to stapedius, occipitofrontalis, posterior belly of digastric and five peripheral branches to the muscles of facial expression including buccinator) and the *nervus intermedius*, which contains *special visceral sensory* (taste via chorda tympani to the anterior two-thirds of the tongue), *general visceral motor* (to the submandibular ganglion via the chorda tympani, for saliva production) and *somatic sensory* (external auditory meatus) fibres. They enter the antero-superior part of the internal auditory meatus and run towards the medial wall of the middle ear where the sensory fibres (subserving taste, and external auditory meatus sensation) synapse; the cell bodies of the motor fibres are in the motor nucleus in the pons and those of the salivatory fibres in the submandibular ganglion peripherally.

A lower motor neurone seventh nerve palsy will not give rise to ptosis as the levator palpebrae superioris muscle is jointly supplied by the third cranial nerve and sympathetic fibres. The tympanic plexus receives a few sensory branches from the geniculate ganglion of the facial nerve, which supply some of the tympanic membrane and external auditory meatus.

8 Temporal lobe abscesses:
A True
B False
C False
D False
E True

Complications of middle ear infections can be thought of in terms of its neighbouring anatomical relations. Thus:
• *Middle ear complications* Hearing loss (both conductive and sensorineural), recurrent ear discharge, facial nerve palsy
• *Anteriorly* Erosion into carotid artery: haemorrhage, septicaemia
• *Postero-inferiorly* Sigmoid sinus thrombosis or thrombophlebitis (thence to cavernous and lateral intracranial venous sinuses)
• *Posteriorly* Cerebellar abscess
• *Superiorly* Temporal lobe abscess (also remember osteomyelitis, subperiosteal abscess, subdural abscess, meningitis, encephalitis)

A temporal lobe abscess may cause hearing loss due to damage to the auditory area in the lateral sulcus of the anterior transverse temporal gyrus. Damage to the lower fibres

of the optic radiation will cause an *upper* quadrantic homonymous hemianopia because the lower fibres in the optic radiation are from the lower part of the retina which represents the upper part of the visual field. A lower quadrantic homonymous hemianopia is unlikely to be caused by a temporal lobe abscess (more likely by a parietal lobe abscess compressing the upper fibres of the optic radiation). Diplopia may also occur by compression of the sixth cranial nerve but is not common. *Peripheral* nystagmus is seen in disorders affecting the semicircular canals or eighth nerve, in which vertigo is often a prominent feature, and *central* nystagmus in cerebellar disease and brainstem lesions, in which vertigo is not so marked. Thus cerebellar but not temporal lobe abscesses may give rise to nystagmus.

9 Phaeochromocytomas:
A True
B True
C True
D True
E True

Ten per cent of phaeochromocytomas are said to be extra-adrenal (the commonest site is the organ of Zuckerland, adjacent to the aortic bifurcation), 10% bilateral, 10% malignant, 10% multiple and 10% associated with other syndromes e.g. Sipple's (MEN II), neurofibromatosis or Von Hippel-Lindau. Noradrenaline is the main catecholamine secreted but a high proportion of adrenaline is thought to favour an adrenal source. Extra-adrenal and multiple tumours are said to be more common in children due to the persistence of the organ of Zuckerland. Sustained hypertension occurs in 50% of cases and paroxysmal hypertension in 50%. Many patients have postural hypotension due to downregulation of the normal sympathetic reflexes involved in blood pressure control, secondary to chronic catecholamine overproduction.

Prior to surgery, patients should receive 2 weeks of α-blockade (such as with

phenoxybenzamine) to normalize blood
pressure and reduce paroxysmal swings,
followed by one week of β-blockade to
prevent cardiac arrhythmias. Blockade
applied in the reverse order will result in
peripheral vasoconstriction and an elevated
blood pressure.

10 Umbilical herniae:

A False
B True
C False
D True
E True

Neonatal umbilical herniae have a low risk
of strangulation, usually resolve spontaneously and rarely require surgery. They are
commonest in black children. In adults they
are uncommon before the age of 40 and
occur as a consequence of raised intra-
abdominal pressure. The hernia usually
contains omentum and transverse colon,
and occasionally small intestine (epigastric
herniae typically contain extraperitoneal
fat). Infection may ultimately give rise to a
faecal fistula. Strangulation is a common
complication in adults.

11 The following are true about the submandibular salivary gland:

A False
B True
C False
D False
E True

The **submandibular salivary gland** is in two
parts: *superficial*, between the mandible and
mylohyoid, and *deep*, between hyoglossus
and mylohyoid. The lateral surface of the
superficial part overlaps the front of the
medial pterygoid insertion and is grooved
posteriorly by the facial artery. The
hypoglossal nerve passes forward on the
lower border of hyoglossus at the level of
the greater horn of the hyoid bone. It is inferior to the deep part of the gland but does
not cross the submandibular (Wharton's)
duct. The nerve *must* be identified

intraoperatively. The lingual nerve is superior to the deep part of the gland and dips
under the submandibular duct.

Adenolymphomas only occur in the
parotid gland because the other salivary
glands do not contain lymphoid tissue. Sixty
per cent of submandibular gland tumours
are benign (80% in the parotid, 20% in the
sublingual glands) most of which are
pleomorphic adenomas. Of the 40% which
are malignant, most are adenoid cystic
carcinomas.

12 The lingual artery:

A False
B True
C True
D False
E False

The **lingual artery** arises from the anterior
aspect of the external carotid artery above
the superior thyroid artery and passes
forwards along the upper border of the
greater horn of the hyoid bone. It passes
deep to hyoglossus and is crossed by the
hypoglossal nerve. It supplies blood to the
entire tongue, the fibrous septum preventing
any significant anastomosis across the
midline. The submandibular gland receives
its blood supply from the facial artery.

13 The following are true about the parotid gland:

A False
B False
C True
D True
E False

The predominantly serous parotid gland is
surrounded by the parotid sheath derived
from the investing layer of deep cervical
fascia. Within the gland is found the facial
nerve superficial to the retromandibular
vein, which is itself superficial to the
external carotid artery. There may also be
preauricular lymph nodes within the gland
substance or just inside the capsule.
Stensen's parotid duct (5 cm long, same

length as Wharton's submandibular duct) pierces buccinator opposite the *third* upper molar tooth to enter the oral cavity opposite the *second* upper molar tooth.

Submandibular gland calculi are more common than parotid calculi because of the more uphill course of Wharton's compared to Stensen's duct, a higher mucous to serous ratio giving rise to thicker secretions, a higher calcium concentration and a larger duct diameter thus allowing for easier radiological identification. Submandibular calculi tend to produce pain which lasts for minutes to hours, in contrast to the pain from parotid calculi which can last hours to days.

Frey's syndrome develops 6 to 9 months after resection and is due to cross regeneration of divided parasympathetic secretomotor fibres into cutaneous sympathetic fibres. This gives rise to the phenomenon of gustatory sweating. Most patients only require antiperspirants although greater auricular nerve avulsion can help in resistant cases.

14 Nerves supplying the external auditory meatus include:

A True
B False
C True
D True
E False

The **great auricular nerve (C2)** supplies the cranial surface of the auricle and a small part of the lateral surface but not the external auditory canal. The canal itself receives its nerve supply mainly from the **auriculotemporal nerve** (anterior one-half) and the auricular branch of the **vagus nerve** (posterior one-half) with a contribution arising from the **facial nerve** via the tympanic plexus (hence providing the anatomical basis for the appearance of herpes zoster vesicles located in this area) but *not* from the glossopharyngeal nerve as this nerve supplies the middle ear mucosa and mucosal surface of the tympanic membrane.

15 The lateral pterygoid muscle:

A True
B True
C True
D True
E False

This muscle is important in understanding the anatomy of the infratemporal fossa. It originates from two heads: the *upper* from the infratemporal surface of the skull and the *lower* from the lateral surface of the lateral pterygoid plate (which form two of the boundaries of the fossa). These heads fuse to insert into the medial end of the head of the mandible and by a few fibres into the capsule and articular disc of the temporomandibular joint. Its action on its own is to allow active opening of the mouth; it also helps in protrusion of the mandible in conjunction with the medial pterygoid muscle. It is supplied by the anterior division of the mandibular nerve (fifth cranial nerve). Within the infratemporal fossa the maxillary artery is superficial and the mandibular, lingual and inferior alveolar nerves are deep to this muscle.

16 Concerning thyroidectomy:

A True
B True
C True
D False
E True

Preoperatively carbimazole is used for up to 2 weeks to achieve euthyroidism. Beta-blockers such as propranolol may also be used to control sympathetic induced symptoms; they also reduce the vascularity of the thyroid gland and reduce peripheral conversion of T_4 to T_3. Postoperatively carbimazole should be continued for 2 days when thyroidectomy is performed for Graves' disease otherwise there is an increased risk of fulminant postoperative hyperthyroidism. Intraoperatively the strap muscles can usually be retracted although they may need to be divided to allow good exposure. The superior thyroid artery is usually ligated as close to the upper pole of the thyroid as possible to avoid damage to the external laryngeal nerve. Postoperative hypocalcaemia may be due to reversal of thyrotoxic osteoporosis, parathyroid bruising or even inadvertent removal of the parathyroid glands. Calcium supplements (orally or intravenously) with or without oral vitamin D may be required if symptomatic.

17 The following are true about the adrenal glands:

A True
B False
C True
D True
E False

The right adrenal gland is overlapped by the inferior vena cava; the left adrenal is not related to this vessel. The right adrenal is pyramidal, the left crescentic in shape. The blood supply is from three sources: inferior phrenic artery, renal artery and directly from the aorta. Venous drainage usually involves just one vein for each gland. The right vein is shorter than the left and enters the vena cava directly. The left adrenal vein enters the left renal vein.

The **adrenal cortex** is derived embryologically from the intermediate mesoderm and has three layers: *zona glomerulosa* (outer) producing mineralocorticoids, *zona fasciculata* (middle) producing glucocorticoids, and the *zona reticularis* (inner) producing the sex hormones. The **adrenal medulla** is derived embryologically from neural crest cells and produces noradrenaline from its precursor dopamine, which is converted to adrenaline by phenyl ethanolamine-N-methyltransferase (PNMT), an enzyme which is induced by cortisol diffusing from the adrenal cortex.

18 The Eustachian tube:

A True
B True
C True
D False
E True

The **Eustachian** or **pharyngotympanic tube** contains both cartilaginous and bony parts in proportions which are reversed compared to the external auditory meatus, thus the ratio of bony to cartilaginous parts of the Eustachian tube is 1:2. The bony part originates from the anterior wall of the middle ear and perforates the petrous temporal bone. It tapers to its narrowest point where the cartilaginous part commences. It gradually enlarges in aperture and the long posterior flange forms the tubal elevation in the lateral wall of the nasopharynx as an inverted 'J', made prominent by the salpingopharyngeus muscle. The bony part is lined by columnar epithelium with no glands, whereas the cartilaginous part is lined by cilia-bearing respiratory epithelium. Contraction of salpingopharyngeus results in elongation of the tubal elevation and thereby assists in opening the Eustachian tube.

19 The posterior triangle of the neck:

A False
B True
C True
D True
E True

The contents of the posterior triangle are given below:

- *Lymph nodes*   Occipital, supraclavicular
- *Nerves*   Accessory (emerges halfway down the posterior border of sternocleidomastoid, lying on levator scapulae and embedded in investing layer of deep cervical fascia); cutaneous branches of cervical plexus
- *Arteries*   Third part of subclavian artery; transverse cervical and suprascapular arteries (branches of the thyrocervical trunk from the first part of the subclavian artery)
- *Veins*   External jugular vein (pierces roof to enter anterior corner of triangle)

20 Thyroglossal cysts:

A True
B False
C False
D True
E True

22 Hirschsprung's disease:

A True
B True
C True
D False
E True

A **thyroglossal cyst** is one of the congenital abnormalities of the thyroglossal tract which represents the passage of the thyroid gland from the foramen caecum of the tongue to just below the hyoid cartilage. The foramen caecum is located between the filiform and vallate papillae of the tongue. The thyroglossal duct may be patent in association with the cyst. They usually occur in the midline, just above or below the hyoid bone and can present at any age, although more often in the first 10 years of life with an equal sex incidence. A thyroglossal cyst may be differentiated from a true thyroid swelling by movement or tugging of the cyst with protrusion of the tongue.

Sistrunk's operation is the procedure of choice, which involves excision of the cyst together with the central portion of the hyoid bone to reduce the risks of recurrence. The procedure is also used to excise a thyroglossal sinus.

21 There is a higher chance of a solitary thyroid nodule being malignant in:

A True
B False
C True
D False
E False

There is a higher chance of a solitary thyroid nodule being malignant if the patient is male, below the age of 40, and clinically has a recurrent laryngeal nerve palsy or dysphagia. There is a lower chance of malignancy if the patient is thyrotoxic. In children the risk of malignancy in a solitary nodule is about 50%. A patient with a multinodular goitre may also have a thyroid malignancy.

Hirschsprung's disease is a condition affecting neonates characterized pathologically by an aganglionic segment of colon. It affects males more commonly than females and 10% of cases have coexistent Down's syndrome. It is the commonest cause of intestinal obstruction in the newborn and presents with delay in passing meconium in the first 24 hours of life together with abdominal distension and bilious vomiting. Investigations include plain abdominal radiography (showing dilated loops proximal to the affected segment) and rectal mucosal biopsy (showing absence of ganglia but the presence of nerve trunks). Rectal washout with normal saline often relieves the acute obstruction, but if this fails colectomy with formation of a colostomy may be required.

23 Concerning radioiodide therapy:

A True
B False
C False
D False
E True

In patients with a *diffuse toxic goitre* in whom medical therapy has failed, radioiodide therapy is a satisfactory alternative in patients over the age of 45 or those under 45 who do not want surgery. It can also be used in patients with a *toxic nodule* (either solitary or as part of a multinodular goitre). It is also of use in patients over 45 with thyrotoxicosis occurring after surgery; younger patients are usually offered medical treatment first to avoid the risks to an unborn foetus. In the treatment of thyroid cancer, it is indicated in *extracapsular disease* and thyroxine replacement must be discontinued 2 weeks before radioiodide therapy begins.

The dose of radioactive ^{131}I given is proportional to the estimated weight of the thyroid gland and a response is usually seen within 6 to 10 weeks. Treatment can be repeated if unsuccessful. Complications include hypothyroidism (about 30% compared to 10% after thyroidectomy), hyperthyroidism, late hyperparathyroidism, and malignancy.

24 The following relate to the thyroid gland:

A False
B False
C False
D True
E False

The thyroid gland consists of two lateral lobes united centrally by an isthmus which lies in front of the second, third and fourth tracheal rings. The left recurrent laryngeal nerve is more likely to lie behind the inferior thyroid artery than in front, whereas on the right there is an equal chance of it lying in front of or behind the artery. The nerves always lie behind the pretracheal fascia and behind the cricothyroid joint.

The ratio between the amount of T_4 produced to T_3 is 10:1. T_4 is the predominant circulating form although T_3 is more potent and 85% is produced peripherally by monodeiodination from T_4. Most of T_3 and T_4 is bound to thyroxine binding globulin rather than albumin. TSH is a polypeptide produced in the anterior pituitary gland after stimulation by thyrotrophin-releasing hormone (TRH) from the hypothalamus. Primary abnormalities of both TSH and TRH are uncommon.

25 Hypercalcaemia:

A False
B True
C False
D True
E False

Malignancy is the commonest cause of hypercalcaemia in hospitalized patients. The commonest primary sites are breast and lung. The metastases associated with prostatic carcinoma are osteosclerotic and hypercalcaemia is rare. Hypercalcaemia due to malignancy may cause a hypochloraemic metabolic alkalosis, in contrast to primary hyperparathyroidism which may cause a hyperchloraemic metabolic acidosis. Symptoms can be improved by simple rehydration, with frusemide added to increase urinary calcium excretion. Disodium etidronate may be used successfully in more severe cases.

Primary hyperparathyroidism may be due to an adenoma (90%), hyperplasia (9%) or a carcinoma (1%) and is characterized by a high serum calcium and low phosphate. Note that secondary hyperparathyroidism occurs in response to hypocalcaemia such that serum calcium may be normal but parathyroid hormone levels are elevated. Radiological investigation may reveal subperiosteal bone resorption on the radial side of the middle and terminal phalanges of the hands, 'pepperpot' skull or cystic bone lesions ('brown tumour'). Preoperatively, patients are warned of recurrent laryngeal nerve injury, the possibility of a failed neck dissection, and of postoperative hypocalcaemia. Surgery for hyperplasia involves removal of three and one-half glands. For parathyroid carcinoma, parathyroidectomy is accompanied by ipsilateral hemithyroidectomy.

ANSWERS TO EXTENDED MATCHING QUESTIONS

Topic: Adrenal hyperfunction

1 A

Cushing's disease is adrenal hyperplasia due to excess ACTH production from the pituitary gland. It is commonest in 30 to 50-year-olds and in women. Surgical treatment directed at the pituitary may be by the transphenoidal or transfrontal approach. Radiotherapy may also be used. Metyrapone can be used as medical treatment. Clinical features are those of Cushing's syndrome which include muscle wasting, osteoporosis, thinning of the skin, bruising, obesity and water retention.

In terms of tests, plasma ACTH is raised (<250 ng/L) and there is no suppression with the overnight dexamethasone suppression test, but some suppression with the high dose dexamethasone suppression test.

2 E

This may indicate ectopic ACTH secretion, most often by a small cell carcinoma of the lung or a bronchial carcinoid tumour. Here, there is no suppression of cortisol with high dose dexamethasone.

3 C

Suppression with prolonged low dose dexamethasone (over 48 hours) is a useful test in distinguishing pseudo-Cushing's syndrome (such as secondary to alcohol abuse or severe depression) from Cushing's syndrome itself, as the latter condition will fail to suppress with this test. The two conditions may be otherwise difficult to diagnose as they both fail to suppress with the overnight or the standard low dose dexamethasone tests.

4 C

Corticotrophin releasing factor is released from the hypothalamus and stimulates the release of ACTH.

Topic: Abdominal pain in children

1 B

Intussusception classically presents at around this age and passage of blood per rectum may follow the initial presentation by 24 hours.

2 A

Although more common in males, congenital hypertrophic pyloric stenosis can occur in females and is often initially detected by increased feeding.

3 F

Although appendicitis is a more common cause of right iliac fossa pain in this age group, the presence of a hypochloraemic microcytic anaemia may indicate loss of blood from a Meckel's diverticulum.

Topic: Inguino-scrotal problems

1 A

The absence of transillumination indicates that the lump is probably solid, and together with the inability to distinguish it as a separate lump from the testis suggests that the most likely option is a testicular tumour.

2 C

This is part of the differential diagnosis of a painful hemiscrotum in a child of this age.

3 E

If at this age a testis can be milked to the fundus of the scrotum it is likely to be retractile. Incompletely descended testes also tend to be smaller than the opposite side.

D: Abdomen

1 In the inguinal region:

A The skin is supplied by the second lumbar spinal nerve

B Direct inguinal hernias are associated with aortic aneurysms

C In females inguinal hernias are more common than femoral hernias

D Division of the ilio-inguinal nerve in the inguinal canal predisposes to direct inguinal hernias

E The inferior epigastric artery is medial to the deep inguinal ring

2 Recurrent inguinal hernias:

A Are more commonly indirect than direct

B Of the direct type usually occur late

C Ischaemic orchitis is more likely after repair of a recurrent inguinal hernia than after primary repair

D Are more common in the presence of postoperative wound haematoma

E With modern techniques of repair recurrence rates at 5 years should be around 5%

3 The following may predispose to gallstones:

A Increased dietary cholesterol

B Increasing age

C Ileal resection

D Clofibrate therapy

E Thyrotoxicosis

4 Femoral hernias:

A Are rare in Africans

B Weight loss is a predisposing factor

C Are more common in patients who have undergone surgery for an inguinal hernia

D Recurrence is higher after repair by the crural than inguinal approach

E The extraperitoneal approach is associated with the highest rate of recurrence compared with other approaches

5 Inguinal hernia repair:

A Should be undertaken in all indirect hernias due to the risk of strangulation

B By the Shouldice method should use braided sutures due to their strength

C Bilateral repair is associated with a higher mortality rate than unilateral repair

D The open mesh repair causes less post-operative pain than the Shouldice repair

E Under local anaesthesia is associated with a lower incidence of deep venous thrombosis

6 Laparoscopic surgery:

A For gallstone disease should not be performed in acute cholecystitis

B Hypothermia is a potential complication

C Intra-abdominal pressure should not exceed 10 mmHg

D The Verres needle is inserted just above the umbilicus

E Acidosis is a complication

7 The oesophagus:

A Is crossed by the right pulmonary artery

B Inclines forwards and to the left at the oesophago-gastric junction

C Blood supply to the cervical part is from the inferior thyroid arteries

D The lower one-third is most easily approached from the left side

E The posterior vagal trunk is more closely applied to the oesophagus than is the anterior trunk

8 The thoracic duct:

A Passes from left to right behind the oesophagus

B Lies anterior to the intercostal branches of the aorta

C Enters the left brachiocephalic vein

D Passes behind the vagus nerve in the root of the neck

E Commences at the level of the 12th thoracic vertebra

9 Gastro-oesophageal reflux:

A Endoscopy is normal in 30% of cases

B Hiatus hernias in patients over 50 are more likely to be asymptomatic than symptomatic

C Dysphagia is a complication of Nissen's fundoplication

D Anti-reflux surgery may reduce the risk of cancer developing in Barrett's oesophagus

E Initial management may include increasing the number of meals eaten per day

10 Achalasia:

A The cause is hypertrophy of the gastro-oesophageal sphincter

B Dysphagia is mainly for solids

C Incidence is higher in males than females

D Manometry shows reduced pressure within the lower oesophagus

E Initial treatment is with H_2 antagonists

11 The azygos vein:

A Receives venous blood from the middle one-third of the oesophagus

B Passes through the aortic opening of the diaphragm

C Receives the left bronchial veins

D Enters the right brachiocephalic vein at the level of T4

E Is joined by the hemiazygos vein

12 Concerning the physiology of gastric motility:

A Circular smooth muscle has a richer innervation than longitudinal muscle

B Gastric emptying is inhibited by secretin

C The lower oesophageal sphincter has a pressure of approximately 30 mmHg

D Fundal contractions are stronger than those originating from the antrum

E Gastric contractions are of a lower frequency than duodenal contractions

13 Tumours of the oesophagus:

A When benign tend to occur in the lower oesophagus

B Are more common at points of physiological narrowing

C Tylosis is a risk factor

D Radiotherapy is the preferred method of treatment for postcricoid tumours

E Are associated with blood group A

14 Appendicitis:

A May present with pain on hip flexion

B Nausea and vomiting are most severe when the appendix is in a pelvic position

C At operation the specimen is sent for histological confirmation of appendicitis

D An appendix mass presenting within 24 hours of onset requires prompt surgery

E Perforation is more common in elderly patients

15 Pancreatic secretion:

A Has a higher sodium concentration than is found in saliva

B The aqueous component has a higher concentration of potassium than plasma

C Contains trypsin inhibitor

D Is inhibited by gastrin

E Approximately 1 litre per day is produced

16 The duodenum:

A A posterior ulcer is more likely to give rise to haemorrhage than an anterior one

B The second part is related to the hilum of the right kidney

C Duodenal ulcers are more common than gastric ulcers

D Has valvulae conniventes throughout its length

E Is partly supplied by the inferior pancreaticoduodenal artery

17 The inferior mesenteric artery:

A Supplies the lateral half of the transverse colon

B Lies anterior to the left psoas muscle

C Becomes the superior rectal artery as it crosses the pelvic brim

D Is beneath the paraduodenal recess

E Is posterior to the body of the pancreas

18 Liver biopsy:

A Is performed through the right sixth intercostal space

B Must not penetrate more than 6 cm beneath the skin

C A haemoglobin less than 10 g/dL is a contraindication

D Can be performed in the presence of ascites

E Is better performed by the transjugular route in sedated patients

19 The hepatic portal vein:

A Commences at the union of the splenic and inferior mesenteric veins

B Has the superior pancreaticoduodenal vein as one of its tributaries

C Lies behind the second part of the duodenum

D Is anterior to the epiploic foramen

E In the porta hepatis is related posteriorly to the hepatic artery

20 In portal hypertension:

A Formation of oesophageal varices may develop if the portal pressure rises above 15 mmHg

B The majority of portal blood bypasses the liver and travels in portosystemic collateral channels

C Primary prevention of bleeding can be achieved with propranolol

D When post-sinusoidal may be secondary to polycythaemia

E Hypokalaemia may precipitate liver failure

21 Complications of gastrectomy include:

A An increased risk of fractures

B An increased incidence of gallstones

C Megaloblastic anaemia

D Steatorrhoea

E Dumping syndrome in most patients

22 Crohn's disease:

A Is associated with ankylosing spondylitis

B Relapse occurs more often in smokers than in non-smokers

C Involving the colon has an increased risk of colorectal cancer

D Is associated with amyloidosis

E Is characterized by mucosal pseudopolyps

23 Colonic adenomas:

A Most are distal to the splenic flexure

B Villous adenomas greater than 3 cm should be treated by laparotomy

C Tubular adenomas are more common than villous

D May give rise to a metabolic acidosis

E Of the villous type are more likely to become malignant than of the tubular type

24 The following are true about colorectal carcinoma:

A There is a correlation between the consumption of meat and animal fat and colon cancer

B The adenomatous polyposis coli (APC) gene is on chromosome 5

C Local spread tends to be in a longitudinal than lateral direction

D Perforation usually occurs through the carcinoma itself

E Hereditary non-polyposis colon cancer accounts for approximately 10% of all cases of colorectal cancer

25 The anal canal:

A Is supplied mainly by the middle rectal artery

B Lymph from the lower canal drains to deep inguinal nodes

C The external anal sphincter has a bony attachment

D Mucosal lining below the pectinate line is derived from endoderm

E Inferior rectal branches of the pudendal nerve supply sensation to the upper half of the anal canal

EXTENDED MATCHING QUESTIONS

Topic: Jaundice

A Cancer of the head of the pancreas
B Alcohol induced cirrhosis
C Porta hepatis metastases
D Cholangiocarcinoma
E Primary sclerosing cholangitis

For each of the cases below, select the most likely cause from the list of options above. Each option may be used once, more than once or not at all.

1 A 27-year-old male with a 7 year history of ulcerative colitis presents with jaundice, lethargy and pain in the right upper quadrant. Investigations reveal a markedly raised alkaline phosphatase, moderately raised aspartate transaminase and bilirubinuria.
2 A 54-year-old male presents with a recent history of anaemia, dark stool and a raised alkaline phosphatase.

Topic: Steatorrhoea

A Coeliac disease
B Chronic pancreatitis
C Tropical sprue
D Alcohol induced hepatitis
E Crohn's disease

For each of the cases below, select the most likely cause from the list of options above. Each option may be used once, more than once or not at all.

1 A 19-year-old woman presented to her GP with pale offensive stools several weeks after returning to the UK from a 3 month trip to Nepal. On examination she was of short stature, with evidence of mouth ulceration and a rash consisting of itchy blisters mainly over her knees and elbows.
2 A 47-year-old man with a history of depression and chronic alcohol intake presents with generalized upper abdominal pains, backache and pale floating stools. He is not jaundiced. Gamma glutaryl transferase is only slightly elevated. Amylase is normal.

Topic: Hepatitis

A Hepatitis A
B Hepatitis B
C Hepatitis C
D Hepatitis D
E Epstein–Barr virus

For each of the statements below, select the most likely virus to which it applies from the list of options above. Each option may be used once, more than once or not at all.

1 An RNA virus spread by blood products.
2 A DNA virus which is a risk factor for hepatocellular carcinoma.
3 This virus is not associated with subsequent malignancy or chronic liver disease.
4 A patient with anorexia, sore throat, splenomegaly and right upper quadrant pain 4 weeks after incubation of this virus.

1 In the inguinal region:
A False
B True
C True
D False
E True

The inguinal canal is an intermuscular space lying above the inguinal ligament. It extends from the **deep inguinal ring** (an opening in the transversalis fascia) to the **superficial inguinal ring** (gap in the medial end of external oblique aponeurosis). The skin over the inguinal region is supplied by the first lumbar root via the ilioinguinal nerve, with a contribution from S2/S3 at the medial end.

The **inferior epigastric artery** is a branch of the external iliac artery just before the inguinal ligament, and after piercing the transversalis fascia crosses the arcuate line to enter the rectus sheath. It is a constant landmark representing the medial relation of the deep inguinal ring, and the lateral relation of the inguinal triangle of Hesselbach. Thus a hernial sac passing lateral to the artery through the deep ring is an *indirect* hernia, one passing medial to the artery through the inguinal triangle is a *direct* hernia.

Inguinal hernias are 10 times more common in males than females. Sixty per cent are indirect, 35% direct and 5% both. They are more common on the right (ratio 5:4). In males they are considerably more common than femoral hernias. In adult females, femoral hernias are more common than inguinal ones although in females of all ages inguinal hernias are slightly more common.

Direct hernias are more common with advancing age. This may in part be due to a collagen defect, either acquired or inherited. They are associated with smoking and aortic aneurysms. The ilioinguinal nerve has a motor supply to the lower fibres of the internal oblique and transversus muscles, which is given off *before* it enters the inguinal canal. Thus division of this nerve within the inguinal canal will not impair flattening of the roof of the canal, and therefore ought not to affect the incidence of direct hernias. It will however cause a sensory loss over the anterior part of the scrotum and thigh. Over half of direct hernias are bilateral.

Strangulation in an inguinal hernia is more common in indirect than direct ones, and is almost twice as likely to occur on the right than left.

2 Recurrent inguinal hernias:
A True
B True
C True
D True
E False

Recurrent inguinal hernias are of the indirect type in 55% of cases and of the direct type in 45%. Indirect recurrences tend to occur early and direct ones late. Recurrence rates should be less than 2% if modern techniques of repair are used. A proportion of recurrences in fact represent a different type of hernia occurring which may have been missed initially. Risk factors for recurrence include sepsis, inexperience of the surgeon, poor operative technique and wound haematoma. Ischaemic orchitis is a complication which is more common following repair of a recurrent than a primary hernia. This is because of thrombosis in the pampiniform plexus. The risk of this complication can be minimized by avoiding dissection medial to the pubic tubercle. Most recover with a scrotal support and do not require antibiotics.

3 The following may predispose to gallstones:
A False
B True
C True
D True
E False

The formation of gallstones revolves around three factors:

1 Supersaturation of bile
   • Increased cholesterol concentration: female sex (oestrogens), increasing age, oral contraceptive, clofibrate
   • Reduced bile salt concentration: ileal resection, cholestyramine
2 Nucleating factors
   • e.g. Bacteria or foreign body
3 Gallbladder stasis
   • Motility of gallbladder reduced by oestrogens, truncal vagotomy, long term parenteral nutrition

Eighty per cent of gallstones are mixed, containing both cholesterol and calcium salts. Twelve per cent are pigment stones and 8% are composed of cholesterol only.

4 Femoral hernias:
A True
B True
C True
D False
E False

Femoral hernias are more than twice as common in females than in males. They are characterized by protrusion of the femoral sac into the femoral canal, which is bounded medially by the lacunar ligament, laterally by the femoral vein, anteriorly by the inguinal ligament and posteriorly by the pectineal ligament and pectineus muscle. The sac usually contains omentum only but occasionally also some bowel. They are rare in Africans.

Predisposing factors include weight loss, multiparity and previous inguinal hernia repair (especially in males). As it enlarges it passes through the fossa ovalis and twists around its tough upper border to extend in an upward and medial direction. Differential diagnosis includes an inguinal hernia, obturator hernia (deeper and more lateral), saphena varix (note that an enlarging femoral hernia can obstruct the saphenous vein by stretching of the cribriform fascia), enlarged Cloquet's lymph node, psoas abscess, femoral aneurysm and an ectopic

testis. The femoral site is the commonest location for development of a Richter's hernia, especially on the right.

The main complication of a femoral hernia is strangulation. Constriction occurs owing to fibrosis of the neck of the sac where it meets the tight anteromedial margins of the femoral canal. Thus femoral hernias should be repaired promptly. There are three main approaches: *crural* (straightforward, often used in elective repairs), *inguinal* and *extraperitoneal* (used in strangulated hernias). Recurrence rates are 15% for the crural and extraperitoneal approaches and 30% for the inguinal. The inguinal approach is also associated with an increased risk of postoperative inguinal hernia although this can be reduced by concomitant repair of the inguinal canal.

5 Inguinal hernia repair:
A False
B False
C False
D True
E True

The Royal College of Surgeons of England published guidelines on the management of different types of groin hernias in adults in 1992. Surgical treatment is recommended in the majority of cases although repair of a small, easily reducible direct inguinal hernia in the elderly is not compulsory. Indirect inguinal hernias should be corrected surgically if they are unsightly or cause pain, or when the risk of subsequent strangulation in the future is deemed to exceed the risks of operative intervention. The risk of strangulation is higher with increasing age, in primary indirect versus direct hernias, when the hernia is irreducible, in right sided hernias and with recurrences which are of an indirect (but not direct) type. This information can therefore help to determine the appropriate timing of surgery.

There are a large number of different methods of repair. The advantages and disadvantages of the main ones are given in Table 4.

Table 4

	Advantages	Disadvantages
Laparoscopic	Less post-op pain and faster return to work than all open methods	Takes longer, thus more expensive
Open mesh repair	Less post-op pain and faster return to work than Shouldice method	Maybe slightly higher incidence of wound complications than Shouldice
Shouldice	Fewer recurrences than other suture methods (Bassini)	More pain, slower return to work than laparoscopic/mesh repairs

The Shouldice repair should use monofilament nonabsorbable sutures as braided ones increase the risk of infection. Simultaneous bilateral hernia repair is not associated with a higher mortality rate although the incidence of scrotal oedema, urinary retention and recurrences may be higher. Thus in the elderly it may be advisable to repair each hernia separately.

Repair under local anaesthesia has the advantages of early postoperative mobilization, fewer urinary complications, lower incidence of deep venous thrombosis and is safer for the patient with severe cardiorespiratory disease. It is contraindicated in the morbidly obese, complicated hernias including those which are strangulated, anxious patients and those who express a desire for a general anaesthetic.

6   Laparoscopic surgery:
A False
B True
C False
D False
E True

Establishing a pneumoperitoneum is performed under general anaesthesia with muscle relaxation. A spring loaded Verres needle with a blunt probe is inserted into the peritoneal cavity via a sub-umbilical stab incision. Approximately 3 litres of CO_2 is usually required for an adult ensuring that the intra-abdominal pressure does not exceed 15 mmHg.

Contraindications include:
• Generalized faecal peritonitis
• Intestinal obstruction with significant bowel dilatation
• Ascites
• Previous abdominal surgery (relative)
• Clotting abnormality

The place of laparoscopic cholecystectomy in the management of acute cholecystitis is controversial. Most authorities recommend conservative management for the acute episode followed by interval cholecystectomy approximately 6 weeks later. However some surgeons perform laparoscopic cholecystectomy during the acute attack. Patients tend to recover much more quickly than if they had been managed conservatively, and do not require another admission in the future. The disadvantage is that the surgery is technically more demanding and takes longer resulting in a slightly higher perioperative morbidity. Thus such surgery should only be considered within 48 hours of the acute attack to minimize these difficulties. Those patients with no other co-morbidity who stand to lose earnings by multiple admissions to hospital may benefit from immediate surgical intervention.

In prolonged operations, gas leakage may allow water to evaporate thereby causing heat loss. Thus hypothermia is a potential complication and core temperature should be monitored. Other complications are given below:

Table 5

	Blood supply	Venous drainage	Lymph drainage
Cervical	inferior thyroid artery	inferior thyroid vein then brachiocephalic	lower deep cervical retropharyngeal
Thoracic	thoracic aorta	azygos	posterior mediastinal nodes
	bronchial artery	hemiazygos	
Distal	left gastric artery	left gastric vein then portal system	left gastric then coeliac nodes
	left inferior phrenic artery		

Secondary to pneumoperitoneum:
- Impaired ventilation due to diaphragmatic splinting
- Ventilation-perfusion shunts
- Deep venous thrombosis (secondary to partial obstruction of inferior vena cava)

Secondary to CO_2 absorption:
- Acidosis
- Sinus bradycardia
- Decreased stroke volume

7 The oesophagus:
A True
B True
C True
D True
E False

The oesophagus begins in continuity with the cricopharyngeus muscle at the level of the cricoid cartilage (C6 vertebra) and is 25 cm (10 inches) long. It lies in front of the prevertebral fascia, and enters the thoracic inlet in front of T1. It descends in contact with the vertebral bodies and occupies a position slightly to the left of the midline, passing behind the left main bronchus and right pulmonary artery. Below this level it begins to incline forwards to pass in front of the descending thoracic aorta. It pierces the diaphragm 2.5 cm to the left of the midline at the level of T10. The intra-abdominal portion measures approximately 1–2 cm and inclines forwards and to the left. As the diaphragm orifice is almost vertical, the posterior wall of the abdominal oesophagus is shorter than the anterior wall.

The anterior vagal trunk is more closely adherent to the anterior surface of the oesophagus than the posterior trunk is to its posterior surface. Both trunks lie slightly to the right of the midline. Lying in the lesser omentum they are known as the nerves of Latarjet. The anterior trunk gives off the large hep atic branch, and the posterior trunk gives off the large coeliac branch.

The blood supply, venous drainage and lymphatic drainage from the different segments of the oesophagus are shown in Table 5.

An oesophageal carcinoma involving the cardia is best approached via a *left* thoracotomy in the sixth intercostal space, and those involving the thoracic oesophagus via a *right* thoracotomy in the fourth or fifth intercostal space (taking care to avoid the azygos vein). Cervical tumours may require pharyngolaryngectomy with or without colonic transposition through incisions in the neck.

8 The thoracic duct:
A False
B True
C False
D True
E True

The **thoracic duct** begins as a continuation of the cisterna chyli at the level of T12. Initially between the aorta and azygos vein it ascends anterior to the right posterior intercostal arteries. In the thorax it passes from right to left posterior to the oesophagus crossing it at the level of T5. It arches over the dome of the left pleura, anterior to the inferior cervical (stellate) ganglion and posterior to the vagus nerve before draining into the origin of the left brachiocephalic vein. In its course it receives lymph from the cisterna chyli, left posterior intercostal nodes, left jugular and left subclavian lymph trunks.

The **right lymphatic duct** receives the right jugular, right subclavian and right bronchomediastinal trunks and drains into the origin of the right brachiocephalic vein either as the main duct or as each trunk separately. Thus the thoracic duct drains all the lymph of the body except from the right arm, right thorax and right side of the head and neck.

9 Gastro-oesophageal reflux:

A True
B True
C True
D False
E True

Gastro-oesophageal reflux may be acidic or alkaline. When *acidic* it is closely associated with inflammation of the lower oesophageal epithelium (oesophagitis). Contributory factors include weakening of the lower oesophageal sphincter (alcohol, smoking, scalds or burns, infection, instrumentation), raised intra-abdominal pressure (pregnancy, obesity), postural or secondary to a hiatus hernia. Oesophagitis leads to vagus nerve overactivity which has two effects: (1) hyperacidity, and (2) longitudinal muscle contraction causing the cardia to be pulled upwards. These two effects both augment oesophagitis, which is made worse in the supine position adopted at night. Thus a vicious cycle is set up. When *alkaline* it may be due to an oesophago-gastro-jejunostomy

without a Roux-en-Y loop.

More than one-third of hiatus hernias occur in people over the age of 50 and in these less than one-third are symptomatic. In patients with proven reflux, 40% of barium swallows, 30% of endoscopies and 20% of mucosal biopsies are normal. In such circumstances, 24 hour ambulatory pH monitoring is indicated. Complications include haemorrhage, stricture formation (occurs in 10%), Barrett's oesophagus (occurs in 10%, results in 30-fold rise in risk of adenocarcinoma), inhalational pneumonitis and obstruction.

Treatment is initially by lifestyle modification (losing weight, stopping smoking, increased frequency and reduced volume of meals, raising the head of the bed, reducing alcohol and caffeine intake) followed by H_2 receptor antagonists, with proton pump inhibitors used in resistant cases. Nissen's fundoplication is successful in 90% of cases. Complications include dysphagia (10%), recurrence or persistence of reflux (5%) and gas bloat syndrome (5%). There is no evidence that anti-reflux surgery reduces the risk of cancer in the presence of Barrett's oesophagus. Alternatives include the Angelchik prosthesis which is reported to have as good reflux control but a higher incidence of dysphagia than surgery.

10 Achalasia:

A False
B False
C False
D False
E False

Achalasia is a rare condition mainly affecting 30–60 year olds characterized by the absence of ganglionic cells in Auerbach's submucosal plexi in the oesophagus. The whole of the oesophagus is aganglionic, in contrast to Hirchsprung's disease in which the aganglionic segment is preceded by a normal colon. Symptoms include pain (from vigorous non-peristaltic contractions), regurgitation, dysphagia worse for liquids than solids, and pneumonitis. Investigations include barium swallow (dilated oesophagus with tapering of distal end – bird's beak) and manometry if radiography is equivocal (absence of peristalsis together with a lower oesophageal sphincter which is non-relaxing and which has a high pressure). Treatment is initially by balloon dilatation. Symptoms are relieved in 70% of cases with up to three attempts being allowed. If unsuccessful, Heller's oesophagomyotomy is performed which involves division of the circular and longitudinal muscle layers only whilst leaving the mucosa intact (similar to Ramstedt's pyloromyotomy but in contrast to a Heineke-Mikulicz pyloroplasty which involves a full depth incision).

11 The azygos vein:
A True
B True
C False
D False
E True

The ascending lumbar and subcostal vein on the right join to form the commencement of the **azygos vein**, at approximately the level of the renal vein. It passes through the aortic opening of the diaphragm and receives blood from the lower right 8 posterior intercostal veins (5–12), middle third of the oesophagus, right superior intercostal and bronchial veins. It enters the superior vena cava at the level of T4.

The **hemiazygos vein** is formed from similar tributaries as the azygos vein but on the left. It ascends through the aortic opening in the diaphragm. It drains the 4 lower left posterior intercostal veins (9–12), entering the azygos vein at T8. The **accessory hemiazygos vein** drains the 4 middle left posterior intercostal veins (5–8) and also receives blood from the middle third of the oesophagus and bronchial veins. It enters the azygos vein at T7.

12 The physiology of gastric motility:
A True
B True
C True
D False
E True

In the stomach the circular smooth muscle layer is thicker than the longitudinal layer, particularly in the antrum. The circular layer is also more richly innervated. These features are in keeping with the predominantly digestive function of the stomach. The fundus is particularly adapted for storage by virtue of its thinner muscular layer and weaker contractions compared with the antrum. This gives rise to the phenomenon of receptive relaxation (mediated by the vagus nerve) whereby intragastric pressure rises considerably less than the increase in volume of stomach contents. This facilitates storage and controlled digestion of food. Hence vagotomy may cause a disproportionate increase in intragastric pressure with only a small rise in volume thereby resulting in dumping. Gastric contractions (3 per minute) are slower than those in the duodenum (10–12 per minute).

Gastric emptying is increased by gastrin and inhibited by duodenal amino acids and peptides (via cholecystokinin), duodenal pH below 3.5 (via secretin) and duodenal hypertonicity.

The lower oesophageal sphincter fluctuates daily around a baseline of about 30 mmHg. Factors which maintain its integrity include the right crus of the diaphragm, oesophago-gastric angle, the intra-abdominal oesophagus (approximately 2 cm) and gastric mucosal folds.

13 Cancer of the oesophagus:
A True
B True
C True
D True
E False

Oesophageal carcinoma represents 5% of all cancers of which the majority are squamous cell and 5% adenocarcinomas. It is 3 times more common in males than in females. In general it occurs most frequently at sites of physiological narrowing, that is at 15 cm (cricopharyngeus constriction), 23 cm (aortic arch), 28 cm (left main bronchus) and 38 cm (oesophageal hiatus in diaphragm) from the incisor teeth. Benign lesions and adenocarcinomas are both more likely to be in the lower oesophagus than elsewhere. Risk factors are as follows:

Those for squamous cell carcinoma

• *Dietary*   Reduced thiamine, proflavine, vitamins A, C, zinc, molybdenum; increased nitrites and nitrosamines
• *Lifestyle*   Smoking, alcohol
• *Oesophageal disorders*   Plummer-Vinson, achalasia, chronic oesophagitis
• *Predisposing influences*   Coeliac disease, tylosis

Those for adenocarcinoma

• Barrett's oesophagus

(Blood group A is associated with gastric carcinoma.) Appropriate and simple initial investigations include full blood count, liver function tests and chest X-ray. More complete staging by mediastinal CT and liver ultrasound may be warranted if the first line tests are normal. Seventy-five per cent of cases are not amenable to curative surgery of which two-thirds may receive some form of palliative therapy such as intubation with an Atkinson or Celestin tube, laser or diathermy or a bypass procedure. Only 25% of cases are potentially curable and surgery is guided by anatomical location and extent. Upper one-third lesions are preferably treated with radiotherapy rather than pharyngolaryngectomy with colon transposition as this allows preservation of the voice and avoids the difficulties of trying to achieve acceptable margins of excision in this part of the neck. Middle one-third lesions are treated by Ivor Lewis oesophago-gastrectomy through upper abdominal and right thoracotomy incisions, or by radiotherapy, and lower one-third lesions by a left thoraco-abdominal approach. In both of the last two cases,

resection is accompanied by Roux-en-Y anastomosis to establish continuity and to stop bile reflux into the lower oesophagus.

14 Appendicitis:

A False
B True
C False
D False
E True

Appendicitis may arise from a primary infection involving the lymphoid tissue of the appendix itself, or secondary to impaction of a faecolith in the appendiceal lumen causing obstruction. In either case luminal oedema ensues which is made worse by progressive venous outflow restriction. If severe enough this leads to arterial obstruction, ischaemia and eventually gangrene. Thus *aetiological factors* include poor diet (reduced fibre slows transit time thereby favouring faecolith impaction and bacterial colonization) and infection (increased bacterial colonization, and lymphoid hypertrophy). The classical presentation of vague visceral periumbilical pain radiating to the right iliac fossa and gradually assuming a constant somatic quality is present in about 50% of patients. Other presentations include profound vomiting and diarrhoea (think pelvic appendix), pain on internal rotation of the hip indicating obturator nerve irritation, hip flexion indicating psoas abscess (note that the hip is most comfortably held in this position) and right upper quadrant pain in pregnancy. Diagnosis can be difficult in young children and women of childbearing age as reflected by the negative appendicectomy rate which is higher in these groups than in men. In elderly patients clinical features can be vague resulting in a high incidence of perforation (>50%) rather than a low negative appendicectomy rate.

A mass in the right iliac fossa if suggestive of an appendix abscess necessitates prompt drainage by ultrasound or CT guided control. However an appendix mass (composed of inflammatory tissue in the absence of any collection) is usually managed conservatively with intravenous antibiotics followed by interval appendicectomy approximately 6 weeks later (Oschner-Sherren regime). At appendicectomy it is usual practice to send the appendix for histological analysis as in less than 1% of cases an underlying carcinoid tumour may be detected. If this is greater than 2 cm or has been incompletely excised, a right hemicolectomy will be necessary. The diagnosis of appendicitis is a clinical one and does not itself require histological confirmation.

15 Pancreatic secretion:

A True
B False
C True
D False
E True

The pancreas produces 1–2 litres of secretions per day. This comprises an *enzymatic component* produced by acinar cells which contains trypsinogen, chymotrypsinogen, procarboxypeptidase, α-amylase, lipases and trypsin inhibitor. Duodenal enteropeptidase activates trypsinogen into trypsin which in turn activates chymotrypsinogen to chymotrypsin and procarboxypeptidase to carboxypeptidase. The *aqueous component* is produced by the ductal columnar cells. It has a higher bicarbonate and lower chloride concentration than plasma, the concentrations of sodium and potassium being similar. Its concentration of Na^+ is higher than that in saliva. This is because the primary saliva produced by the salivary acini (similar in composition to plasma) is modified in the ducts such that Na^+ and Cl^- are resorbed in exchange for K^+ and HCO_3^-. The low NaCl concentration thereby lowers the threshold of the taste receptors for salt.

Pancreatic juice is released in response to three well described phases: *cephalic* (vagus nerve), *gastric* (via gastrin and free amino acids) and *intestinal* (via acidic chyme in the duodenum stimulating secretin release, and fat stimulating cholecystokinin release) phases. Secretin augments the aqueous bicarbonate containing content, and cholecystokinin the enzyme content of pancreatic juice.

16 The duodenum:

A True
B True
C True
D False
E True

The **duodenum** is 25 cm long (same as the oesophagus and the ureter) and is divided into 4 parts (see Table 6).

The first 2 cm of the first part of the duodenum is smooth and does not have any valvulae conniventes. The blood supply to the duodenum is from the superior pancreaticoduodenal artery (from the coeliac trunk) and the inferior pancreaticoduodenal artery (from the superior mesenteric artery). The gastroduodenal artery, a branch of the hepatic artery, passes posterior to the first part of the duodenum to the left of the common bile duct. Thus a posterior duodenal ulcer is more likely to lead to haemorrhage than an anterior one. Duodenal ulcers are 4 times more common than gastric ulcers.

Table 6

	Length (cm)	Surface marking	Important associated structures
1st	5	L1	IVC, epiploic foramen (post.)
2nd	7.5	L2	Hilum R kidney (post.)
3rd	10	L3	Aorta (post.), pancreas (sup.), crossed by SMA/SMV
4th	2.5	L2	Left psoas muscle (post.), DJ flexure and ligament of Treitz

17 The inferior mesenteric artery:

A False
B True
C True
D False
E False

Arising from the anterior surface of the aorta at the level of L3 the inferior mesenteric artery passes posterior to the third and fourth parts of the duodenum. It crosses over the left psoas, sympathetic chain and left common iliac artery and is medial to the left ureter. The inferior mesenteric vein lies lateral to it. On crossing the pelvic brim it becomes the superior rectal artery. It supplies the left one-third of the transverse colon, descending and sigmoid colon and the rectum to the dentate line of the anus. It is smaller than the superior mesenteric artery. The inferior mesenteric vein is associated with the paraduodenal recess and can be found just lateral to the ligament of Treitz.

18 Liver biopsy:

A False
B True
C True
D True
E True

Liver biopsy is usually performed through the right eighth or ninth intercostal space in the midaxillary line. This is because the right border of the liver extends from the sixth to tenth ribs and costal cartilages, thus entry into the sixth space may miss the liver. The needle must not penetrate more than 6 cm from the skin otherwise the inferior vena cava may be entered. Patient co-operation is required for percutaneous liver biopsy. Transjugular biopsy may be used in sedated patients. It has the advantage of not causing intraperitoneal haemorrhage or biliary peritonitis.

Contraindications to percutaneous liver biopsy include anaemia (Hb<10g/dL), abnormal clotting, low platelet count (<100 × 10^9/L), hydatid cyst, haemangioma or in the presence of bile duct obstruction. *Relative contraindications* include adhesions, perihepatic collections and ascites; biopsy in these situations can still be performed but is safer under ultrasound control.

19 The hepatic portal vein:

A False
B True
C False
D True
E True

The **hepatic portal vein** is formed from the splenic vein and superior mesenteric vein at the level of the junction of L1 and L2. It passes upwards behind the first part of the duodenum before entering between the two layers of the lesser omentum. It ascends in its free edge with the hepatic artery in front and to the left, and the bile duct lying in front and to the right of the vein. These structures form the *anterior* margin of the aditus to the lesser sac (epiploic foramen of Winslow), *posteriorly* being the inferior vena cava, *superiorly* the caudate process of the liver and *inferiorly* the first part of the duodenum.

Other than the two main veins from which it originates, it has as direct tributaries the right and left gastric veins and the superior pancreaticoduodenal veins. The other veins draining the remainder of the gastrointestinal tract enter into either the splenic, superior or inferior mesenteric veins.

20 In portal hypertension:

A True
B True
C True
D True
E False

The portal venous pressure should normally be less than 10 mmHg; when greater than 15 mmHg oesophageal varices may form. Causes include:

• *Pre-hepatic* (20%) Portal vein thrombosis, compression by porta hepatis lymph nodes

• *Hepatic* (80%)   Cirrhosis, schistosomiasis, multiple metastases
• *Post-hepatic* (rare)   Constrictive pericarditis, tricuspid regurgitation, Budd-Chiari syndrome (may be spontaneous, or associated with oral contraceptive, polycythaemia or malignancy)

The risk of a first bleed is 30%, but once bleeding has occurred, 70% of these will rebleed. Propranolol is a β-blocker used to reduce portal venous pressure. The severity of the hepatic disease is assessed according to Child's classification or its modification outlined by Pugh, each of which incorporate 5 parameters: serum bilirubin, albumin, ascites, encephalopathy and the nutritional state (Child) or prothrombin time (Pugh). The severity of each of these parameters combines to give an overall grade from A (least severe) to C (most severe). It is used in the assessment of prognosis and fitness for anaesthesia.

In portal hypertension 80% of portal blood is shunted into portosystemic collateral channels (lower end of oesophagus, upper end of anal canal, bare area of liver, periumbilical region and retroperitoneum) leaving only 20% to reach the liver. However this adaptive response does not appreciably reduce the degree of hypertension. Hepatic encephalopathy may be precipitated by electrolyte abnormalities especially hypokalaemia (although this does not by itself precipitate liver failure), infections, GI bleeds and drugs including pethidine.

21 Complications of gastrectomy include:
A True
B True
C True
D True
E False

Complications can be *early*, such as haemorrhage from the anastomotic line, paralytic ileus, stomal obstruction or pancreatitis. *Late* complications include post-gastrectomy syndromes (see below), anastomotic ulcers, gastrojejunocolic fistula (presents as severe

diarrhoea in a patient following a gastrojejunostomy) or carcinoma in the gastric remnant.

Postgastrectomy syndromes occur in about 20% of patients and can be subdivided as below:

Postcibal

• Early dumping (high osmotic content in duodenum reduces plasma volume causing postural hypotension)
• Late dumping (surge of insulin causing hypoglycaemia)
• Bilious vomiting

Nutritional

• Weight loss and malnutrition
• Steatorrhoea (rarely, following colonization of a blind loop or due to decreased biliary or pancreatic flow)
• B_{12} deficiency (more common than folate deficiency, due to lack of intrinsic factor and due to gastric mucosal atrophy secondary to bile reflux)
• Osteomalacia and osteoporosis (normal bone ageing is advanced; also minor degrees of vitamin D deficiency are recognized)
• Gallstones (note: although patients with ileostomies have an increased incidence of renal stones, this association has not been shown after gastrectomy)

22 Crohn's disease:
A True
B True
C True
D True
E False

Crohn's disease is a chronic granulomatous inflammatory condition which occurs most commonly in 15–30-year-olds although any age can be affected. The sex distribution is equal. It is more common in Jews and Caucasians. Both types of inflammatory bowel disease are associated with HLA B27 and ankylosing spondylosis. Macroscopic pathological examination shows deep fissures and ulcers producing cobblestoning, and discontinuous skip lesions affecting any part of the gastrointestinal tract although the terminal ileum is involved in 70% of patients. Microscopically, transmural inflammation and non-caseating granulomas occur in approximately 50%. Note that ulcerative colitis has twice the prevalence of Crohn's, has its peak incidence between the ages of 30 to 40, is slightly more common in females and is characterized by regenerative mucosal pseudopolyps, crypt abscesses and mucosal inflammation.

The *risk of colorectal carcinoma* in inflammatory bowel disease is in proportion to the extent and duration of disease, but is only appreciable for pan-colitis with more than 10 year disease. It presents at a younger age and tumours may arise anywhere in the colon and are commonly multiple, in contrast to sporadic cancers which tend to be left sided.

Extra-intestinal associations include amyloidosis (rare), aphthous ulcers, finger-nail clubbing, pyoderma gangrenosum, arthritis and sacro-ileitis, uveitis and renal oxalate stones. Hepatobiliary complications include cholelithiasis, fatty change of the liver, cholangiocarcinoma and sclerosing cholangitis.

23 Colonic adenomas:
A True
B True
C True
D True
E True

Polyps are swellings arising from proliferated epithelium and contain a fibrovascular core. They may be pedunculated if they possess a stalk, or sessile if they grow directly from the bowel wall. Occurring in the gastrointestinal tract the majority are found in the colon. Adenomas may cause rectal bleeding or intussusception. Tubular adenomas are more common than the villous type, the latter being more common in females and on account of their propen-

sity to produce large quantities of potassium-rich mucus, may give rise to hypokalaemia and if severe a metabolic acidosis.

All adenomas carry the potential for malignancy, especially if multiple, greater than 2 cm diameter, villous in type and in the presence of cytological atypia on histology.

Polyps are removed by diathermy snaring although sessile ones may be excised locally. Inaccessibility, more than 3 cm in size or malignancy on histology are indications for laparotomy.

24 The following are true about colorectal carcinoma:
A True
B True
C False
D False
E True

Direct lateral spread is more common than in the longitudinal direction. Intramural spread distal to the lesion is particularly important in rectal cancer where it rarely exceeds 1 cm. Thus traditional resection margins for clearance need not be greater than 2 cm.

Perforation as a complication of colorectal cancer may occur through the lesion itself, but more commonly occurs distal to it. The commonest example of this is caecal perforation secondary to a closed loop obstruction where the ileocaecal valve is competent.

Most colorectal cancers arise as a consequence of the polyp-cancer sequence, except those in ulcerative colitis which arise directly from colonic epithelial dysplasia. Predisposing factors include the Western diet (high animal, low vegetable fat, low fibre, high beer), inflammatory bowel disease, familial adenomatous polyposis (FAP) and hereditary non-polyposis colorectal cancer (HNPCC).

FAP accounts for 1% of colorectal cancers. It is autosomal dominant. Cancer usually occurs by the age of 30, and requires prophylactic colectomy with formation of ileo-anal pouch or subtotal colectomy with ileorectal anastomosis and frequent screening of rectal mucosa. The APC gene is located on chromosome 5.

HNPCC accounts for 10% of cancers. It is also autosomal dominant. It mainly results in right sided lesions. Cancer usually occurs by the age of 50. The gene is linked to chromosome 2.

Other polyposis syndromes are Gardner's and Peutz-Jeghers.

25 The anal canal:
A False
B False
C True
D False
E False

The lining of the upper half of the anal canal is embryologically derived from endoderm, and that of the lower half from ectoderm. The dividing line is considered to be at the pectinate or dentate line, which is at the level of the anal valves. This division is important for blood and nerve supplies and lymph drainage. The main blood supply to the upper anal canal arises from the superior rectal artery (from the inferior mesenteric artery) and that to the lower canal from the inferior rectal artery (a branch of the internal pudendal artery, itself a branch of the anterior division of the internal iliac artery). There is a rich anastomosis to which the middle rectal artery contributes a little. Sensory supply to the lower half of the canal is from somatic inferior rectal branches of the pudendal nerves (S2), whereas autonomic nerves pass to the upper half where pain is not felt. Lymph drainage from the upper half is to internal iliac nodes, that from the lower half to superficial inguinal nodes.

The external anal sphincter has three parts although these blend into one another to a degree: *deep* (blends with levator ani), *superficial* (attaches to tip of coccyx posteriorly and perineal body anteriorly) and *subcutaneous* (circular ring just below the lower end of the internal sphincter) parts. It is supplied by the pudendal nerve, whereas the internal sphincter is supplied by autonomic fibres.

ANSWERS TO EXTENDED MATCHING QUESTIONS

Topic: Jaundice

1 D

This is associated with inflammatory bowel disease even at a young age. Sclerosing cholangitis is a possibility although it is not usually primary.

2 C

The most likely possibility is a metastatic gastrointestinal malignancy (such as from a gastric or right sided colonic primary) causing gradual blood loss.

Topic: Steatorrhoea

1 A

The most likely options are either coeliac disease or tropical sprue. The presence of itchy red blisters on her knees and elbows is suggestive of dermatitis herpetiformis which is associated with coeliac disease. The recent foreign travel is therefore not relevant.

2 B

The options here are between B and D. In the absence of jaundice and markedly deranged liver function tests, acute hepatitis is less likely. The history fits more with chronic pancreatitis. Amylase is often normal in this condition owing to destruction of a significant proportion of the pancreatic tissue.

Topic: Hepatitis

1 C

2 B

3 A

4 E

E: Urology

MULTIPLE CHOICE QUESTIONS

1 Antidiuretic hormone:

A Is released in response to a reduced glomerular filtration rate

B Secretion is reduced by atrial natriuretic peptide

C Causes vasoconstriction

D Secretion is enhanced by increased stimulation of low pressure volume receptors in the left atrium

E Increases permeability of the collecting duct to urea

2 The following factors encourage potassium movement into cells:

A β-blockers

B Aldosterone

C Acidosis

D Reduced plasma osmolality

E Reduced dietary potassium

3 Renal calcium excretion is increased in the presence of:

A Alkalosis

B Reduced parathyroid hormone levels

C Reduced extracellular fluid volume

D Hypophosphataemia

E Chronic renal failure

4 Organ transplantation:

A Hyperacute rejection occurs due to ABO incompatibility

B Tissue matching is rarely performed in heart transplantation

C Of the liver can be from a live related donor

D Of the bone marrow does not require ABO compatibility testing

E The maximum permissible cold ischaemic time varies according to the warm ischaemic time in renal transplantation

5 Wilm's tumour:

A Is more chemoresistant than renal cell carcinoma

B Is bilateral in 10% of cases

C Is associated with exomphalos

D Is associated with macroglossia

E Rarely present with an abdominal mass only

6 Renal cell carcinoma:

A Smoking is a risk factor

B Mainly affects proximal tubular cells

C Pyrexia of unknown origin is a recognized mode of presentation

D May cause hypertension

E Tonsillar metastases are recognized

7 Urological investigations:

A Delayed films on intravenous urography are indicative of obstruction

B Ultrasound demonstrates function better than plain X-ray

C Creatinine tends to underestimate the measurement of *GFR*

D A DTPA scan with captopril can help to distinguish renal artery stenosis from chronic pyelonephritis

E DTPA scanning is better than DMSA for assessing renal scarring

8 The following increase sodium reabsorption in the proximal convoluted tubule:

A ACE inhibitors

B Activation of the sympathetic nervous system

C Aldosterone

D Increased *GFR*

E Increased hydrostatic pressure in the peritubular capillaries

9 The following factors reduce renal blood flow:

A Adrenaline

B Indomethacin

C ACE inhibitors

D Atrial natriuretic peptide

E Dopamine

10 Aldosterone:

A Secretion may be stimulated by a low serum potassium concentration

B Excess may be produced by hyperplasia of the zona fasciculata of the adrenal cortex

C Causes vasoconstriction

D Its action is antagonized by amiloride

E Excess may cause alkalosis

11 The anion gap:

A Reflects the unmeasured plasma anions

B Is increased in hyperalbuminaemia

C Is increased in renal failure

D Is decreased in hypercalcaemia

E Is decreased in hyperphosphataemia

12 Transitional cell carcinoma:

A About 60% of superficial (Stage Ta and T1) bladder tumours will recur after resection

B Schistosomiasis is a risk factor

C Of the upper urinary tract should be followed up postoperatively by regular check cystoscopies

D On presentation may have infected urine in one-third of cases

E Invasive tumours are usually treated either by cystectomy or chemotherapy

13 Urinary stone disease:

A Cystinuria can be treated by penicillamine

B Urate stones are radiolucent

C Frusemide administration is a predisposing factor

D Calcium phosphate are the commonest type

E Is more common in patients with ileostomies

14 Pelvi-ureteric junction (PUJ) obstruction:

A May be idiopathic

B May be secondary to tuberculosis

C May be associated with methysergide administration

D May respond to steroids

E Can be confirmed by retrograde ureterogram

15 The kidney:

A Lies anterior to the lateral cutaneous nerve of the thigh (roots L2, L3)

B Renal hila are situated at the level of the transpyloric plane

C The right renal artery is shorter than the left

D The renal pelvis is the most posterior of the three main structures at the hilum

E Develops from the mesonephros

16 The ureter:

A On the left lies lateral to the inferior mesenteric vessels

B Is crossed by the genitofemoral nerve

C On the right is crossed by the superior mesenteric vessels

D Receives part of its blood supply from the middle rectal artery

E Innervation by sympathetic fibres is responsible for initiation of peristalsis

17 The following are more common after renal transplantation:

A Hypertension

B Gynaecomastia

C Gingival hyperplasia

D Atherosclerosis

E Gout

18 The following are true about congenital kidney abnormalities:

A Absence of a kidney is more common on the right

B Horseshoe kidney is associated with an increased risk of trauma

C Horseshoe kidney is more common than pelvic kidney

D Pelvic kidney is more common in males

E Renal vascular anomalies are more common in pelvic kidneys

19 Regarding the innervation of the bladder:

A The detrusor muscle is supplied by parasympathetic fibres

B The pudendal nerve is partly responsible for maintaining continence

C Abolishing sympathetic input to the bladder prevents normal bladder emptying

D Spinal cord transection above S2 would cause abnormal distension of the bladder 6 months after injury

E In a cauda equina lesion at S4, abnormal distension of the bladder would gradually resolve once the initial phase of spinal shock passes

20 Benign prostatic hypertrophy:

A Tends to affect the outer zone of glandular tissue

B Is characterized pathologically by nodular hyperplasia

C May present with hydronephrosis

D Is premalignant

E TURP is indicated in all cases of acute retention associated with an enlarged prostate on digital rectal examination

21 Adenocarcinoma of the prostate:

A Causes more deaths per year than colorectal cancer

B The fascia of Denonvilliers temporarily slows anterior spread

C Prostatic acid phosphatase is a better marker for extracapsular spread than prostate specific antigen

D Diagnosis is more accurate in the presence of acid mucin

E Grade 2 has more cellular polymorphism than grade 4

22 The male urogenital region:

A The deep perineal pouch contains the external urethral sphincter

B The superficial perineal pouch contains the spermatic cords

C The perineal membrane is attached to the ischiopubic rami

D Rupture of the membranous urethra would cause urine extravasation into the anterior abdominal wall

E The urogenital diaphragm is attached to the anococcygeal body

23 The testis:

A Descends into the scrotum just before birth

B Lymphatic drainage is to the inguinal nodes

C Is incompletely descended if it comes to rest in the superficial inguinal pouch

D Has the epididymis on its posteromedial surface

E The left testicular vein may join the inferior vena cava

24 Testicular tumours:

A Cryptorchidism gives rise to tumours which are more likely to be seminomatous than non-seminomatous

B Teratomas are more common than seminomas

C Ectopic testis has a higher risk of subsequent malignancy than maldescended testis

D Spread in seminomas is usually blood borne

E Mumps may be a risk factor

25 CAPD:

A Is the recommended form of dialysis in diabetic patients

B Peritonitis is mainly caused by staphylococci

C Is less likely to give rise to anaemia after long term use than haemodialysis

D Intra-abdominal adhesions are a contraindication

E Is recommended in the elderly

EXTENDED MATCHING QUESTIONS

Topic: Urological malignancy

A Radical nephrectomy
B Radical prostatectomy
C Nephroureterectomy
D Transurethral resection of the prostate
E Hormonal manipulation
F Chemotherapy

For each of the patients below, select the single most appropriate initial treatment from the list of options above. Each option may be used once, more than once or not at all.

1 A 60-year-old man presents with haematuria. Investigations reveal a transitional cell carcinoma of the renal pelvis.
2 An 80-year-old man presents with a weak urinary stream and localized skeletal pain. His serum prostate specific antigen level is 800 ng/mL. Prostatic biopsies confirm the presence of a Gleason grade 3+4 adenocarcinoma. A bone scan reveals bony lesions consistent with metastatic disease. He initially undergoes TURP for obstructive symptoms.
3 A 59-year-old man presents with an adenocarcinoma of the prostate. The Gleason grade is 1+2, the stage is T1M0. He has no obstructive symptoms.

Topic: Renal transplantation

A 2 haplotype match
B 1 haplotype match
C No DR mismatch, and 0–1 mismatches at A and B loci
D No DR match
E 0 haplotype match

For each of the statements below, select the single most appropriate antigen match from the list of options above. Each option may be used once, more than once or not at all.

1 In any one family, 50% of siblings would be expected to have this match.
2 One-year graft survival of 95% can be achieved with this match in an unrelated or cadaveric transplant.
3 One-year graft survival of 95% can be achieved with this match in a live related transplant.
4 In a cadaveric transplant, 1-year graft survival would not be expected to be more than 60%.

Topic: Renal calculi

A Percutaneous nephrostomy
B Extracorporeal shock wave lithotripsy (ESWL)
C Alkalinization of the urine
D Non-steroidal anti-inflammatory analgesia
E Double J stent

For each of the statements below, select the single most appropriate therapy from the list of options above. Each option may be used once, more than once or not at all.

1 A 24-year-old man has a 4 mm stone present in the lower one-third of his right ureter.
2 A pregnant woman develops pyelonephritis secondary to a stone visualized in the middle one-third of her right ureter. She is pyrexial.
3 A 55-year-old man presents with right loin pain and microscopic haematuria. He had a pacemaker fitted 2 years ago following a myocardial infarction, and is known to have a stable 4 cm abdominal aortic aneurysm. A 9 mm stone is present at the junction between the upper and middle third of the right ureter. There is no proximal obstruction and he is apyrexial.
4 This treatment may be used for a radiolucent stone.

ANSWERS TO MULTIPLE CHOICE QUESTIONS

1 Antidiuretic hormone:
A True
B True
C True
D True
E True

Antidiuretic hormone or vasopressin is a 9 amino acid protein produced in the supraoptic nuclei of the hypothalamus and transported axoplasmically to the posterior pituitary. From there it is released in response to a change in blood osmolality or volume. Hypothalamic osmoreceptors can detect a change in osmolality of less than 1% whereas a change in blood volume of 5–10% is required to result in ADH release. Volume receptors exist in the left atrium (low pressure) and carotid sinus and aortic arch (high pressure). ADH release is inhibited by alcohol and by atrial natriuretic peptide (ANP). In the normal diuretic state, due to the medullary gradient, water is still reabsorbed in the collecting duct, mainly in the lower part. In the antidiuretic state, the effect of ADH is to increase the permeability to water of the cortical part of the collecting duct. Thus in the presence of ADH more water is absorbed cortically and less in the medullary collecting system. It also increases the permeability of the medullary collecting duct to urea.

2 The following factors encourage potassium movement into cells:
A True
B True
C False
D True
E True

Potassium movement into cells is encouraged by insulin (co-transport mechanism), catecholamines acting via α receptors (but not via β_2 receptors which inhibit it), aldosterone, alkalosis and reduced osmolality (water enters cells which lowers the intracellular K^+ concentration, thus K^+

enters to maintain electroneutrality). Reduced dietary potassium results in increased K^+ reabsorption in the distal convoluted tubule.

3 Renal calcium excretion is increased in the presence of:
A False
B False
C False
D True
E True

Renal calcium excretion is increased in acidosis, hypophosphataemia, reduced parathyroid hormone levels (such as follows hypercalcaemia), chronic renal failure and an expanded extracellular volume. Contraction of the extracellular fluid volume increases Na^+ and water reabsorption by the proximal tubule, thereby enhancing Ca^{2+} reabsorption by passive solvent drag and *reducing* its excretion.

4 Organ transplantation:
A True
B True
C True
D True
E True

Hyperacute rejection occurs as a result of antibodies to the ABO group which are already present, or to Class 1 HLA molecules which have been acquired from either previous blood transfusion, pregnancy or a previous graft. *Acute vascular rejection* occurs within 3 months of the transplantation and occurs as a result of antibodies which may not have been detectable during the initial crossmatch but which rise in titre due to memory cell activation. *Acute rejection* may begin as soon as 5 to 7 days after transplantation and is due to a cell mediated T-cell response. *Chronic rejection* involves multiple mechanisms including immune complex deposition, antibody mediated response, viral infection of graft or recurrence of the original disease. In heart and liver transplantation, tissue matching is usually impossible because of the small donor pool. The liver is less aggressively rejected than other organs. In bone marrow transplants, T-cell rejection is more important than antibody-mediated. ABO blood group compatibility and the serological crossmatch do not matter, but HLA tissue typing is vital. There is also the additional risk of graft versus host disease. In renal transplantation, the *warm ischaemic time* is usually about 1 to 2 minutes, the maximum being 30 minutes. The maximum *cold ischaemic time* is about 72 hours but this depends on a short warm ischaemic time; thus if the latter is prolonged, the maximum tolerated cold ischaemic time is shorter.

5 Wilm's tumour:
A False
B True
C True
D True
E False

Wilm's tumour is bilateral in 10% of cases and is inherited on chromosome 11. It is associated with aniridia, hemihypertrophy, exomphalos and macroglossia. It is treated in specialized paediatric oncology centres by nephrectomy, radiotherapy and chemotherapy. They are more chemosensitive than renal cell carcinomas.

6 Renal cell carcinoma:
A True
B True
C True
D True
E True

Risk factors for **renal cell carcinoma** include male sex, smoking, increasing age, chronic haemodialysis, caffeine and occupational contact with cadmium, lead and asbestos. It is also associated with Von Hippel-Lindau syndrome (cerebellar and retinal angiomas). The tumours are usually polar and result from proliferation of proximal tubular cells

which demonstrate glycogen in their cytoplasm. Less than 10% present with the classical triad of loin pain, palpable mass and haematuria. Other modes of presentation include non-specific features such as pyrexia of unknown origin, raised ESR, anaemia and amyloidosis. Paraneoplastic effects may occur due to hormone secretion by the tumour, including hypertension, polycythaemia and hypercalcaemia. Left sided varicocele may occur due to tumour compression of the left testicular vein. Metastases may cause bone pain or masses in unusual places such as the tonsil, or may result in vena cava obstruction.

7 Urological investigations:
A True
B False
C False
D True
E False

Intravenous urography demonstrates more detailed anatomy than on plain X-ray, shows up filling defects in the urinary tract, and gives an indication of kidney function if contrast excretion is delayed or absent. **Ultrasound** can differentiate between solid and cystic masses but gives no information about function. It can also guide needle biopsies. **Isotope renography** (DMSA, dimercaptosuccinic acid or DTPA, diethylene triamine pentacetic acid) is used as a measurement of renal function. DMSA is taken up by tubules, thus its uptake is proportional to renal plasma flow. Hence it is good for measuring differential *GFR* (better than DTPA). It is also better than DTPA at demonstrating kidney scarring. DTPA is not taken up by the tubules as much and is instead eliminated. Thus it is very good at measuring urinary flow and obstruction. The ACE inhibitor captopril causes more vasodilatation in the efferent compared to the afferent glomerular arterioles. Hence captopril administration in the presence of renal artery stenosis will cause a profound drop in perfusion pressure to the glomerulus and a concomitant change in the

DTPA scan. Creatinine is filtered at the glomerulus and subsequently secreted into the proximal convoluted tubule, thus it tends to overestimate the true glomerular filtration rate.

8   **The following increase sodium reabsorption in the proximal convoluted tubule:**
A   False
B   True
C   False
D   True
E   False

Angiotensin II stimulates sodium and water reabsorption in the proximal tubule. Thus ACE inhibitors will have the opposite effect. **Aldosterone** stimulates NaCl reabsorption by the distal convoluted tubule and collecting duct but not the proximal tubule. The **sympathetic nervous system** enhances NaCl and water absorption in the proximal tubule, thick ascending limb of the loop of Henle, distal tubule and the collecting duct. An increased GFR results in an increased filtered load of sodium presented to the proximal tubule. As a constant proportion of sodium is reabsorbed here, this means that a greater quantity of NaCl is reabsorbed when the GFR rises (called glomerulotubular balance). This is part occurs because an increased GFR results in an increased peritubular osmotic pressure, thus setting up the Starling forces in favour of enhanced sodium and water reabsorption. Likewise an increased hydrostatic pressure in the peritubular capillaries (such as due to a reduced GFR) will inhibit sodium reabsorption.

9   **The following factors reduce renal blood flow:**
A   True
B   True
C   False
D   False
E   False

Factors which reduce renal blood flow include catecholamines (adrenaline,

noradrenaline), antidiuretic hormone and non-steroidal anti-inflammatory agents. Dopamine, ACE inhibitors and ANP all increase renal blood flow.

10 **Aldosterone:**
A   False
B   False
C   False
D   True
E   True

Aldosterone is produced in the zona glomerulosa of the adrenal cortex. It is secreted in response to an increase in plasma angiotensin II concentration, or hyperkalaemia. Its effects are to increase serum sodium thereby bringing about expansion of the extracellular volume and hypertension, and to reduce serum potassium which may in turn give rise to an alkalosis. It is not a vasoconstrictor. Amiloride antagonizes its action in the principal cells of the distal tubule, and also inhibits sodium reabsorption directly.

11 **The anion gap:**
A   True
B   True
C   True
D   True
E   False

The **anion gap** is derived from the formula $AG = (Na^+ + K^+) - (Cl^- + HCO_3^-)$. In other words it is the measured cations minus measured anions, or conversely the unmeasured anions minus unmeasured cations. It therefore reflects unmeasured anions of which albumin is the major constituent (others include phosphate, sulphate, lactate). Thus hyperalbuminaemia will increase the AG. Other conditions which are associated with an *increased AG* include metabolic acidosis, renal failure, diabetic ketoacidosis, lactic acidosis and salicylate overdose. Conditions associated with a *reduced AG* include hypoalbuminaemia, paraproteinaemia and hypercalcaemia (increased unmeasured plasma cation).

12 Transitional cell carcinoma:
A True
B False
C True
D True
E False

Transitional cell carcinomas are almost all malignant, low grade and well differentiated. They arise from the urothelial surface epithelium and have a propensity for synchronous or metachronous lesions due to field change. Risk factors include male sex, smoking and occupational related aromatic amines (2-naphthylamine). Schistosomiasis and chronic bladder irritation or infection are risk factors for squamous cell carcinoma. Haematuria is the main symptom although in one-third of cases there may be infected urine on presentation. Ten per cent present without macroscopic haematuria. About 60% of new bladder tumours are superficial, of which the same proportion will recur after treatment. Thus regular check cystoscopies are mandatory. Upper urinary tract lesions are often treated by nephroureterectomy but postoperative cystoscopy is required to detect for metachronous lesions. Invasive tumours are treated by radical cystectomy or radiotherapy.

13 Urinary stone disease:
A True
B True
C True
D False
E True

Risk factors for urinary stones include male sex (except struvite or magnesium ammonium phosphate stones which are more common in women), hot climate, dehydration, infections, drugs (e.g. frusemide which increase urinary calcium excretion), various metabolic conditions (including hyperparathyroidism, and hyperoxaluria secondary to gut resection or ileostomy formation) or structural stasis (e.g. hydronephrosis, prostatic hypertrophy,

neurogenic bladder, tumours, pregnancy or catheterization). Calcium stones are the commonest type (mixed oxalate/phosphate more common than oxalate or phosphate alone) which are radio-opaque as are struvite stones. Calcium phosphate stones may be treated with thiazide diuretics, low calcium diet and urinary acidification. Cystine stones (semi-opaque) are treated with hydration, penicillamine and urinary alkalinization.

14 Pelvi-ureteric junction obstruction:
A True
B True
C False
D False
E True

Pelvi-ureteric junction (PUJ) obstruction is a cause of unilateral hydronephrosis. It may be *idiopathic* (due to congenital PUJ stenosis, or muscular deficiency in wall of ureter) or *secondary* to infections (e.g. tuberculosis), previous surgery, tumours in the renal pelvis or trauma. It can be confirmed by retrograde ureterography. Methysergide administration is associated with retroperitoneal fibrosis which may benefit from steroids.

15 The kidney:
A False
B True
C False
D True
E False

The kidney develops from the mesoderm in the intermediate cell mass. The *metanephros* ultimately becomes the kidney. The lateral cutaneous nerve of the thigh is too low to be a *posterior relation* of the kidney; the ilioinguinal and iliohypogastric nerves are found posterior to the kidney as are the subcostal neurovascular bundle, quadratus lumborus muscle, 12th rib and diaphragm. *Anterior relations* include the second part of the duodenum (right) and the tail of the pancreas (left), and the hepatic flexure of colon on the right and splenic flexure on the left. The **renal hila** are situated anterior to psoas and are at the level of L1 through which passes the transpyloric plane of Addison. In the hilum the pelvis is posterior to the renal artery which is posterior to the renal vein. The left renal artery is shorter than the right, the latter crossing behind the inferior vena cava.

16 The ureter:

A True
B False
C True
D True
E False

The **ureter** is 25 cm long. In the *abdomen* it lies on the medial border of psoas and runs down over the tips of the lumbar transverse processes. It crosses the pelvic brim over the bifurcation of the common iliac artery. The *right ureter* is crossed by the duodenum, and gonadal, right colic, ileocolic and superior mesenteric vessels. The *left ureter* lies lateral to the inferior mesenteric artery and is crossed by the gonadal and left colic vessels. Both ureters cross the genitofemoral nerve. In the *pelvis* the ureters are crossed by the vas deferens in the male and uterine artery in the female. **Blood supply** comes from a number of sources: the *intra-abdominal* part from branches of the renal, gonadal and common iliac vessels, the *pelvic* part from branches of the inferior and superior vesical and middle rectal arteries. The blood supply to the intra-abdominal part enters the ureter from its medial side, thus it should be mobilized laterally; to the pelvic part it enters the ureter laterally, which should therefore be mobilized medially. Although the ureter has sympathetic input from T11–L2 segments, these are not essential for initiation or propagation of peristalsis. They may contribute to the sensation of pain.

17 The following are more common after renal transplantation:

A True
B False
C True
D True
E True

Long term complications of transplantation include accelerated atherosclerosis, skin cancer, gingival hypertrophy, gastritis (owing to uncoated steroid use), osteoporosis, hypertension (due to renal artery stenosis), cataracts, ureteric stenosis (especially with acute tubular necrosis) and gout. Gynaecomastia is associated with chronic renal failure but not post-transplantation *per se*.

18 The following are true about congenital kidney abnormalities:

A False
B True
C False
D True
E True

Horseshoe kidney, congenital absence of a kidney and pelvic kidney are all more common in males. Pelvic kidney occurs in approximately 1 in 100 people, with horseshoe kidney less common (1 in 400). Congenital absence is more likely on the left than right, whereas pelvic kidney is more common on the right than left. Both horseshoe and pelvic kidney are more prone to trauma, and may be associated with renovascular abnormalities.

19 Regarding the innervation of the bladder:

A True
B True
C False
D False
E False

The detrusor muscle is a functional syncytium formed from a complex interlinking of muscle fibres. Functionally this allows the bladder to increase in volume without an increase in tension, up to a point. Under normal conditions, the bladder is therefore highly compliant. The detrusor is innervated by parasympathetic fibres from the intermediolateral nuclei of S2, 3 and 4. The external sphincter mechanism contains both smooth and striated muscle and is innervated by the perineal branch of the pudendal nerve (also S2, 3 and 4). At rest the intra-urethral pressure exerted by the sphincter comfortably exceeds the intravesical pressure thus favouring continence. Involuntary contraction of the bladder by the detrusor muscle is accompanied by voluntary relaxation of the external sphincter mechanism thereby allowing micturition. Sympathetic fibres exist in the male to innervate the internal urethral sphincter but this acts to prevent seminal reflux during ejaculation and is not involved in urinary continence. The bladder itself does receive sympathetic innervation which may help to carry pain impulses centrally.

Following the initial phase of spinal shock, a *suprasacral cord lesion* above S2 would ultimately give rise to a bladder which would be able to fill and contract reflexly (mediated by the sacral parasympathetic segments S2, 3 and 4) but which would be without central control of the external sphincter mechanism subserved by the rostral pons. Thus there results loss of co-ordination between detrusor contraction and sphincter relaxation, in which the bladder develops high pressures together with infections and upper tract damage. A lesion affecting the *S4 sacral segment* would result in a paralysed detrusor muscle causing the bladder to become abnormally distended. This would persist after the initial phase of spinal shock has passed (which itself gives rise to an overdistended bladder). Overflow incontinence would then follow.

20 Benign prostatic hypertrophy:

A False
B True
C True

D False
E False

Benign prostatic hypertrophy affects the inner zone of glandular tissue. It is characterized histopathologically by hyperplastic smooth muscle and glandular tissue which may have a nodular appearance. It is not thought to be premalignant. *Obstructive* symptoms such as poor stream and hesitancy tend to occur early. In response to outflow obstruction there occurs bladder muscle hypertrophy and trabeculation. Increased detrusor instability may result giving rise to a group of *irritative* symptoms (urgency, frequency, nocturia) which tend to occur later. If the rise in detrusor pressure does not overcome the outflow obstruction, residual urine volume increases which predisposes to further complications such as infection, stone formation, and hydronephrosis ultimately leading to renal failure. **Transurethral resection of the prostate (TURP)** is commonly performed but may not be technically possible if the prostate is too large, or if the patient is unable to adopt the position required for TURP to proceed (e.g. due to osteoarthritis of the hips). In such cases, retropubic prostatectomy may be considered.

21 Adenocarcinoma of the prostate:

A False
B True
C True
D True
E False

The sites most frequently causing cancer death in males in order of decreasing frequency are lung, colorectal, prostate, pancreas and stomach. In females the most common cancer deaths occur from lung, breast, colorectal, ovary and uterus (remember however that skin cancer is much more prevalent than any of the above but does not kill as many people). The *rectovesical fascia of Denonvilliers* is a condensation of connective tissue between the rectum and bladder which may temporarily slow the anterior spread of cancer from the prostate. An elevated **acid phosphatase** is suspicious of extracapsular disease but may occur following recent surgery, instrumentation or acute retention. Also up to 25% of patients with metastatic disease have a normal acid phosphatase. Despite its limitations it is a better marker than **prostate specific antigen (PSA)** for metastatic disease. PSA is a highly sensitive marker with a high rate of false positives in benign disease. It is best used as a marker for assessing response to treatment. Diagnosis is aided by prostatic biopsy or transurethral resection chippings. The **Gleason** grading system ranges from 1 to 5 depending on the degree of differentiation of nuclear and architectural features. Grade 1 represents low grade well differentiated tumour, grade 5 a high grade anaplastic poorly differentiated tumour without tubule formation. It ascribes two scores, one to the predominant pattern and one to the next most common pattern of tumour visualized. The combined score (e.g. 2 + 3 = 5, or 4 + 4 = 8) correlated better with prognosis. Grade 2 has a lesser degree of cellular pleomorphism than grade 4. Diagnosis can be aided by immunohistochemistry: the presence of acid mucin and the absence of a second layer of basal cells increase the accuracy of diagnosis of adenocarcinoma.

22 The male urogenital region:
A True
B True
C True
D False
E True

The **deep perineal pouch** is bounded by the superior and inferior fasciae of the urogenital diaphragm, the inferior one commonly called the perineal membrane. It is divided into 6 layers and contains the external urethral sphincter, membranous part of urethra, deep transverse perineal muscles, perineal branch of the pudendal nerve and pudendal vessels. The **superficial perineal pouch** is bounded by the perineal membrane, and the superficial perineal fascia of Colles. It contains the penile urethra, superficial transverse perineal muscles, scrotal contents, root of the penis and arteries to the penis. The superficial perineal fascia of Colles is a continuation of the membranous layer of superficial fascia (Scarpa's) in the anterior abdominal wall. Rupture of the penile urethra may cause urine extravasation to extend into the anterior abdominal wall. The urogenital diaphragm comprises the external urethral sphincter and the deep transverse perineal muscles, within the deep perineal pouch. It extends from the ischiopubic rami (also the origin of the perineal membrane) to the anococcygeal body.

23 The testis:
A True
B False
C False
D False
E False

At around 4 months of development the testis lies close to the deep inguinal ring, by the seventh month it is in the deep ring, and by birth 80% of testes have descended into the scrotum. The testes should be in the scrotum by 1 year of age but around 3% are not. A testis which is in its correct anatomical path but has not reached the scrotum by birth is *incompletely descended*. A testis which has descended to an abnormal anatomical site is *ectopic*. Examples of ectopic sites include the superficial inguinal pouch, femoral triangle, base of penis and perineum.

The **lymphatic drainage** of the testis is via nodes situated along the testicular artery, to para-aortic nodes lying at the level of origin of the testicular arteries (L2). The overlying scrotal skin drains to the medial group of superficial inguinal lymph nodes. The **left testicular vein** invariably joins the left renal vein; the right testicular vein usually drains directly into the inferior vena cava but may join the right renal vein on occasions. The **epididymis** is on the *posterolateral* surface of the testis.

24 Testicular tumours:
A True
B False
C True
D False
E True

Testicular tumours are classified into *germ cell tumours*, comprising **seminomas** (which make up 40% of all testicular tumours) and non-seminomatous germ cell tumours or **teratomas** (30% of total). *Non-germ cell tumours* include malignant lymphoma which makes up 7% of all testicular tumours, and other rarer varieties including yolk sac tumours. Pathogenesis is thought to include cryptorchidism (failure of testicular descent), genetic factors (lower risk in some black Africans, higher in the UK and USA), testicular dysgenesis and possibly mumps. *Cryptorchidism* gives rise to testicular atrophy followed by dysplasia and malignancy which tends to be seminomatous. It is present in 10% of cases of testicular tumours. The risk is even greater for ectopic than incompletely descended testes. The contralateral testis is also at risk and orchidopexy does not eliminate the risk but permits earlier detection. Teratomas occur at a slightly younger age than seminomas. Characteristically teratomas exhibit blood-borne spread and seminomas lymphatic spread. Blood-borne spread is rare in seminomas.

25 CAPD:
A True
B True
C True
D True
E True

Continuous ambulatory peritoneal dialysis (CAPD) is recommended in children to avoid regular needling, in diabetics as it can help with control of blood glucose stability and in the elderly to avoid hypertensive episodes associated with haemodialysis. It is less likely to give rise to anaemia and peripheral neuropathy after long term use than haemodialysis. CAPD-related peritonitis is mainly due to staphylococci of which the majority respond successfully to antibiotics. Coliform peritonitis is associated with a poorer prognosis. Repeated infections may reduce the adequacy of ultrafiltration in some patients. Postoperative intra-abdominal adhesions make siting of the Tenckhoff catheter more difficult and reduce the subsequent efficiency of dialysis. Thus alternative methods of dialysis should be sought.

ANSWERS TO EXTENDED MATCHING QUESTIONS

Topic: Urological malignancy

1 C

2 E
This man needs hormonal manipulation to control symptomatic bony secondaries.

3 B
This man is potentially curable and thus may benefit from aggressive surgical intervention.

Topic: Renal transplantation

1 B
In a family, 25% of siblings would be expected to have a 2 haplotype match, 50% a 1 haplotype match and 25% no haplotype match.

2 D
In cadaveric or unrelated transplants, it is very rare to have haplotype matching. The aim is to match as many of the DR, A and B alleles as possible. Matching for DR is the most advantageous in terms of graft survival, followed by B then A. One-year graft survival of 90–95% can be achieved with a 'beneficial match' which comprises no DR mismatch and up to one mismatch at the A and B loci.

3 A
Live related transplants give better graft survival than unrelated or cadaveric grafts. For a 2 haplotype match, 1-year graft survival approaches 95%, 1 haplotype match 80% and 0 haplotype match 60%.

4 E
A cadaveric transplant with no DR match has a poor prognosis, with 50–60% graft survival at 1 year.

Topic: Renal calculi

1 D
Ninety-five per cent of stones less than 5 mm in size situated within 5 cm of the vescico-ureteric junction will pass spontaneously within 5 days.

2 A
This lady needs decompression of her proximal urinary tract prior to definitive management of her stone. This is best and most easily achieved by percutaneous nephrostomy.

3 E
Pacemakers and abdominal aortic aneurysms are contraindications to ESWL. In his case the best treatment would be insertion of a double J stent, following which the stone would either pass spontaneously or its removal aided by a dormia basket.

4 C
Urate stones are radiolucent for which allopurinol and urinary alkalinization are the treatments. Cystine stones can also be treated by alkalinization but they tend to be more radio-opaque.

Index